# Harold Shipman's clinical practice 1974–1998

A review commissioned by the
Chief Medical Officer

*I will use my power to help the sick to the best of my ability and judgement; I will abstain from harming or wronging anyone by it. I will not give a fatal draught to anyone if I am asked, nor will I suggest any such thing.*

From the Hippocratic oath.

# Foreword

In January 2000 Harold Shipman, a general practitioner in Hyde, Greater Manchester was convicted of murdering 15 of his patients and of forging the will of one.

These terrible crimes, tragedies for the patients and families concerned, led to widespread feelings of horror and outrage amongst the British public and within the medical profession itself.

The events in Hyde were particularly shocking because they struck at the bond of trust which exists between doctors and their individual patients and which is at the heart of good medical practice throughout the world.

When the nature of Harold Shipman's activities became public knowledge there was particular concern that there may have been other suspicious deaths.

For this reason, as part of the Government's response to the Shipman trial verdict, I was asked by the Secretary of State to conduct a review of his past practice.

This is the report of the review. It has been carried out for me by Professor Richard Baker of the Clinical Governance and Research and Development Unit in the Department of General Practice and Primary Health Care, University of Leicester. Professor Baker has carried out this major task painstakingly, thoroughly and with great skill and rigour. It is not the role of a clinical review of this kind to investigate in detail the circumstances of individual suspicious deaths. Those are matters for the police and other legal authorities. Rather the clinical review examined trends, patterns and clinical decisions in Harold Shipman's practice and compared the data against the practice of his peers (other general practitioners working in the same areas at the same time).

Twenty-four years of Harold Shipman's practice have been reviewed. The clinical review reveals clear evidence of a higher level of deaths than would have been expected, and not just in the most recent of those years. The excess of deaths does not appear to be explicable on grounds that his practices served populations with markedly different demographic or health profiles.

The main excess of deaths is amongst elderly women patients but in some years higher than expected numbers of deaths were found for older men and women in their late 60s. Compared to deaths in neighbouring practices deaths amongst Harold Shipman's patients showed clustering to particular times of day. The clinical review also examined samples of his medical records and cremation forms. Here too irregularities and inconsistencies were found between the clinical history, the circumstances of the death and the certified cause of death.

The analysis, objective and scientific as it is, makes chilling reading. Taken in the round, the clinical review suggests that there must be serious concerns about deaths of some patients during Harold Shipman's entire career as a general practitioner. These must now be investigated by the proper legal authorities.

The questions raised by the report will be distressing reading for the patients and relatives who were under Shipman's care over the years but it is important for their sake that this work has been done and is published. It has started the process of addressing the many unanswered questions that remained after the trial of Harold Shipman had concluded.

Everything points to the fact that a doctor with the sinister and macabre motivation of Harold Shipman is a once in a lifetime occurrence. That does not mean that we should dismiss the need for action beyond the investigation of the events themselves. There is much to be learned from this tragedy. The first duty of a health service is to protect patients from harm. This report is a vital step in that process.

I would like to thank Professor Baker for undertaking this major piece of work which is without precedent.

**Professor Liam Donaldson**
**Chief Medical Officer**

The audit was undertaken by Richard Baker, Professor of Quality in Health Care and Director of the Clinical Governance Research & Development Unit, Department of General Practice & Primary Health Care, University of Leicester. Professor Baker wrote the report and is wholly responsible for its contents and conclusions.

Some assistance was provided with particular aspects of the audit:

Dr Peter Goldblatt, Chief Medical Statistician, Office For National Statistics, co-ordinated the identification of death notifications and organised the prospective audit.

Professor David Jones, Professor of Medical Statistics. Department of Epidemiology & Public Health, University of Leicester, provided advice on the statistical analysis.

From the Department of General Practice and Primary Health Care, University of Leicester,

Dr Robert McKinley, Senior Lecturer, and Dr Andrew Wilson, Senior Lecturer, undertook an independent review of samples of clinical records.

Dr Margaret Stone, Research Associate, contributed to database management.

Dr Ahmed Nana assisted in the review of cremation registers.

December 2000

# Acknowledgements

The audit was commissioned by Professor Liam Donaldson, Chief Medical Officer for England. The field work undertaken to collect data during the audit was facilitated by the assistance of a large number of people, including staff in pharmacies and crematoria, Health Authorities and general practices. Too many individuals assisted to mention them all by name, but two particular groups deserve special mention. First, Greater Manchester Police who allowed access to the information they had collected during their investigations. Without their support, it would have been much more difficult to distinguish the features typical of the murders committed by Harold Shipman. I am particularly grateful to Detective Superintendant Bernard Postles and Detective Inspectors David O'Brien and David Heap. Second, Drs Hannan, Lloyd and Wilson, and the health care team of The Surgery in Market Street, Hyde, gave invaluable help, in particular in undertaking a review of the care of people with diabetes or angina.

I am grateful to Professor Robin Fraser of the Department of General Practice and Primary Health Care, University of Leicester, for his support throughout the audit and for helpful comments on an early draft of the report. I also thank Vicki Cluley for her patience in preparing successive versions of the manuscript.

Guidance was sought from Tameside and Glossop Local Research Ethics Committee on the need for formal ethical approval. Since the data were to be used in an audit and patients would not be identified, formal approval was judged not to be required.

# Contents

# Summary

Following Harold Shipman's conviction for the murder of fifteen of his patients, an audit of his clinical practice from 1974 to 1998 was commissioned by the Chief Medical Officer for England. The aims of the audit were to identify:

(a)     the pattern of observed to expected deaths in particular age groups

(b)     deaths showing unusual clusters in time

(c)     deaths showing unusual clusters by place of death

(d)     the relationship between certified cause of death and medical history

(e)     the integrity of records

(f)     the prescribing of restricted drugs.

In investigating the pattern of deaths, two sources of information were used. In the first, all medical certificates of cause of death (MCCDs) issued by Shipman from 1974 were identified. In order to estimate the number of deaths that would have been expected, those MCCDs issued by a comparison group of local general practitioners who worked during a similar period to Shipman were also identified. Information about the numbers of patients registered with each practitioner was used to calculate the death rates in different age groups of male and female patients.

In the second method of investigating patterns of deaths, a prospective audit was undertaken of the deaths of all patients who were registered with Shipman for any period from 1987. Patients of Shipman were identified from the Health Authority register, and deaths from the National Health Service Central Register. The expected number of deaths among Shipman's patients was estimated from the numbers of deaths in equivalent patient populations based on figures from the local district (Tameside), a group of districts sharing similar population socio-economic characteristics, and figures for England and Wales.

The relationship between certified cause of death and medical history was investigated by review of surviving clinical records and cremation forms. The analysis was strengthened by comparing cremation forms completed by Shipman with those completed by the group of comparison practitioners. The record review was also used to assess the integrity of records, supported by review of the audit trail on a duplicate copy of Shipman's practice computer system.

The prescribing of restricted drugs was investigated through review of data provided by the Prescription Pricing Authority and inspection of the controlled drugs registers at pharmacies in Hyde.

Several methods were used to investigate the pattern of deaths. The findings of review of MCCDs showed that:

•       Shipman issued a total of 521 MCCDs, 499 whilst he worked in Hyde. The highest number issued by any of the six comparison practitioners in Hyde was 210

- The comparison of the numbers of MCCDs issued by Shipman and general practitioners in the same locality with similar patients indicated that he issued an excess total number of MCCDs of 297 (95% confidence interval 254 to 345) and an excess related to deaths occurring at home (including practice premises) of 236 (95% confidence interval 198 to 277)

- The excess was greatest among females aged 75 or above, second highest among females aged 65–74, and third highest among males aged 75 or above

- The excess numbers were evident from the first few years of Shipman's career as a general practitioner

- Six deaths certified by Shipman occurred on practice premises, one in the group practice and five in the single-handed practice.

The prospective audit that included all patients registered with Shipman from 1987 indicated a lower number of excess deaths. The excess was 98 among females 1987–1998, with 12 less than expected among males. Since all patients were included in this analysis, whether or not their illnesses were being directly managed by Shipman, it was probably less sensitive to variations in the annual numbers of MCCDs issued by Shipman.

The review of clinical records and cremation forms suggests that the excess related to deaths at home (236) is most likely to reflect the true number of deaths about which there should be concern. Between 1985 and 1998, information from records and/or cremation forms was available for 288 (88.9%) of the 324 deaths for which Shipman issued MCCDs. 166 (57.6%) of these were classified as highly suspicious and 43 (14.9%) as moderately suspicious on the basis of the relationship between cause of death as certified by Shipman and medical history, and other features typical of the convictions (Shipman present at or shortly before death, death at home, cause of death). The total excess number of deaths between 1985 and 1998 as estimated from the excess among deaths at home was similar – 199.

The review of the audit trail disclosed a small number of records that contained back-dated entries, but it was not possible to judge the integrity of records made on paper. Shipman's standard of record keeping was poor.

The review of cremation forms indicated that in comparison with the other local practitioners:

- Death was more likely to occur in the afternoon

- Be certified as due to heart conditions, stroke or old age

- More likely to occur within 30 minutes and the mode of death being described as syncope or collapse

- Shipman was more likely to be present at the death of his patients, and relatives or carers were less likely to be present.

It was not possible to identify abnormal prescribing of restricted drugs, other than the irregularities already identified by Greater Manchester Police. It is not clear, therefore, how Shipman obtained all the diamorphine necessary.

The findings from the various components of the audit have dreadful implications, and give rise to grave concerns about the activities of Harold Shipman during his career as a general practitioner. It is the duty of health services and health professionals to protect patients from individuals such as Shipman. Therefore, recommendations have been made about arrangements to monitor the death rates of patients of general practitioners, the information collected for death certification, the regular review of general practice records and recording of information about restricted drugs.

# One: Introduction

## 1.1 Aims of the audit

In January 2000 Harold Shipman was convicted of the murder of fifteen patients in his care, and of forging the will of one. The day following the pronouncement of the verdict, the Secretary of State for Health announced arrangements for an Inquiry in order to identify factors that may have enabled these events to occur. The House of Commons was informed that the Crown Prosecution Service was considering further charges and that the police had, at that stage, investigated a total of 136 cases.

In addition to the Inquiry, several other steps were announced. These included:

(i)     plans to require doctors to disclose criminal convictions and steps taken against them by a professional regulatory body, whether in the UK or abroad, before they could be appointed to medical lists;

(ii)    plans to require general practitioners to report deaths in their surgeries and other serious incidents to Health Authorities;

(iii)   a review of death certification procedures and the checks undertaken before cremation and burial;

(iv)    a clinical audit of Shipman's past practice, commissioned by the Chief Medical Officer.

This report describes the methods of the audit, and details the findings and principal implications.

The key aims of the audit were to identify:

(a)     the pattern of observed compared to expected deaths in particular age groups

(b)     deaths showing unusual clusters in time

(c)     deaths showing unusual clusters by place of death

(d)     the relationship between certified cause of death and medical history

(e)     the integrity of records

(e)     the prescribing of restricted drugs.

## 1.2 Shipman's professional career

Shipman graduated from Leeds University Medical School in 1970 (an outline of his career is included in Appendix 1). Following pre-registration hospital posts, he worked in junior hospital posts until 1974, when he became a GP assistant in Todmorden, West Yorkshire. After one month as an assistant, he was invited to become a principal.

However, the partnership was dissolved towards the end of 1975 because Shipman was found to be signing prescriptions for pethidine although the patients were not receiving the medication. He admitted to abusing pethidine, and was convicted of dishonestly obtaining drugs, forgery of an NHS prescription, and unlawful possession of pethidine. He was fined and ordered to pay compensation to the local Family Practitioner Committee.

He then worked as a clinical medical officer in south west Durham, but returned to work as a general practitioner in October 1977, when he joined a group practice in Hyde, Greater Manchester. He remained in that practice until 1992, when he set up a single-handed practice in the same town, and with the same list of registered patients.

In March 1998, Dr Reynolds, a general practitioner from the neighbouring Brooke Practice contacted Stockport coroner to report concerns about the apparent excess numbers of deaths among Shipman's patients. Dr Reynold's concern had been reinforced by suspicions expressed independently by a local undertaker, and by discussion with her partners in the practice. The coroner asked Greater Manchester Police to undertake a confidential investigation that included a review of some clinical records. This initial investigation did not uncover any evidence to substantiate the concerns. In July 1998, the daughter of a patient who had died the previous month contacted the police to report her strong suspicions that her mother's alleged will was a forgery. The suspect will assigned the deceased patient's estate to Shipman. A detailed police investigation commenced, culminating in Shipman's arrest. Consequently, Shipman ceased clinical practice on 7th September, 1998.

The audit is concerned with Shipman's career in general practice from 1974 to 1998.

## 1.3 The Audit Report

To introduce the audit of patterns of deaths, the findings of investigations already conducted are summarised in Section Two and an overview is presented of the numbers of deaths certified by Shipman throughout his working life as a general practitioner. Although this information does not fully describe and explain the observed patterns, it does, however, clarify the issues to be addressed before conclusions may be drawn about whether rates of death were higher among Shipman's patients, and the potential explanations for any observed excess of deaths.

The characteristics of the group of patients registered with Shipman are among the factors that will influence the observed numbers and patterns of deaths. For example, if Shipman's registered list included high proportions of elderly or economically disadvantaged patients, a higher rate of death would be expected. Therefore, in Section Three of the report, the characteristics of Shipman's patients are described and compared with the patients of other Hyde general practitioners.

In subsequent Sections, information is presented to enable a more complete interpretation of the observed patterns of death of Shipman's patients. Section Four deals with documentary evidence from clinical records about care provided by Shipman to those who died. The cases for which Shipman was convicted are briefly considered in order to establish the features typical of the murders. In addition to the content of clinical records, details are drawn from the evidence presented in court. The transcript of the summing up of the case delivered between 10th-21st January 2000 by the Honourable Mr Justice Forbes has been used as the source of information about the trial. Having established the features typical of the murders of which Shipman was convicted, evidence was sought to indicate the presence or absence of these features in other deaths. Much of this evidence was contained in the surviving clinical records. Section Four also includes a discussion of the relationship between certified cause(s) of death and medical history, and the quality and integrity of Shipman's records.

A review of cremation forms completed by Shipman and a comparison group of practitioners is reported in Section Five. The forms contained brief information about the circumstances of death and enabled the identification of cases that shared some of the features characteristic of the convictions.

Section Six reports the findings of a review of the records of the Stockport coroner and Section Seven considers available evidence about Shipman's prescribing of diamorphine and other restricted drugs. During his trial, it was established that Shipman used diamorphine to murder patients. In Section Eight, evidence collected from medical certificates of cause of death issued by general practitioners is presented that describes the patterns of deaths among Shipman's patients between 1974 and 1998 in comparison with deaths among patients of other local practitioners.

Section Nine presents the findings of a prospective audit of the deaths of all those patients who were registered with Shipman from 1987 onwards. In Section Ten the conclusions are outlined, and some preliminary recommendations made in Section Eleven.

# 1.4 Methodological Issues

Clinical audit is *the systematic critical analysis of the quality of care* (Department of Health, 1989). It incorporates a cycle of activities that includes the collection of data to assess performance, the implementation of changes to improve care when necessary, and the collection of data for a second time to determine whether performance has improved (Fraser et al, 1998). Since the implementation of change and a second data collection cannot form parts of the present investigation, the audit is restricted to the first assessment of performance.

The sources of data were those clinical records, certificates and registers relating to the deaths of Shipman's patients since 1974. Clinical judgement has been used to interpret these documents, and inevitably many records from the 1970s and 1980s are no longer available. Furthermore, I have only drawn on information that is documented or can be verified by similar means, and not included informal information given personally by many of those I met during the completion of the audit. Information provided by witnesses to the events in question cannot be explored appropriately within the context of an audit, and are properly matters to be considered by the Inquiry. Thus, the audit cannot precisely determine the circumstances of death of any individual to the level that would be expected in a criminal investigation.

I have sought to present the findings as clearly as possible, and hope that those relatives and friends of Shipman's patients who wish to know what happened find the report helpful. In the interests of clarity, a standard format has been followed to report each component study:

- Background

- Methods

- Findings

- Conclusions.

The audit includes extracts from the clinical records and cremation forms of Shipman's patients. Recent guidance from the General Medical Council (GMC, 2000) on the confidentiality of patient information makes clear that non-anonymised data for clinical audit should not be disclosed without patient consent. Personal information should also be kept confidential after a patient's death, and the extent of any disclosure should depend on the circumstances, including the nature of the information, whether the information is already public knowledge or can be anonymised, and the intended use of the information. The publication of properly anonymised case studies as part of National Confidential Enquiries or other clinical audit would be unlikely to be regarded as improper by the GMC.

In accordance with this guidance, and in order to protect the confidentiality of deceased patients, names, ages and dates relevant to their histories have been omitted. Each patient is referred to by a code number unique to the audit. Information about a small number of general practitioners is also included in the audit. They are also referred to by a number, and information that might suggest their identities has been omitted.

# Two: Background

## 2.1 Introduction

Several investigations of the patterns of deaths of patients of Shipman have already been undertaken, and they are briefly summarised below. In addition, a preliminary summary is presented of the numbers of deaths certified by Shipman from 1974 to 1998.

## 2.2 The Police Investigation

Concerns were raised at an early stage that Shipman might have murdered a large number of patients. Following initial reports that Greater Manchester Police were investigating the deaths of some of Shipman's patients, anxious friends and relatives reported additional cases and these were also investigated. The police used a scoring system to classify deaths according to the likelihood of being able to confirm murder:

- whether the body had been buried;

- whether the family were concerned about the circumstances of death;

- whether the police had cause for concern, for example the certified cause of death not being consistent with the medical records;

- whether the records had been altered.

The police used this system to enable them to concentrate their efforts on cases in which the possibility of conviction would be greatest. However, some cases that did not fulfil these criteria were investigated, and convictions were eventually achieved even when the body had been cremated.

At the conclusion of their investigations in May 2000, the police had made enquiries about 192 deaths. Shipman was convicted of the murder of 15 of these, but the police believed murder was possible in a further 24. In two further cases prosecution was regarded as not in the public interest, as the patients were already suffering from terminal illnesses.

Evidence about another 86 cases was regarded by the police as insufficient for prosecution. The remaining 69 were regarded as not being suspicious. Following Shipman's conviction, the Stockport coroner ordered inquests into the deaths of an additional 26 former patients, including the 24 regarded by the police as having sufficient evidence to obtain conviction. In the inquests completed by October 2000, all three patients were pronounced as unlawfully killed.

## 2.3 The investigation by West Pennine Health Authority

Hyde is situated in the Tameside district of West Pennine Health Authority. The Authority was established in 1994 from Oldham, Glossop and Tameside districts, and in 1998/9 had contracts with 104 general practitioners in Tameside. The principal hospital serving Tameside is Tameside General Hospital (Tameside and Glossop Acute Services NHS Trust), Community services are provided by Tameside and Glossop Community and Priority Services NHS Trust. Following Shipman's arrest, staff at West Pennine Health Authority undertook three reviews of the deaths of Shipman's patients, using the sources of data available to the Authority.

From 1997, those Health Authorities that choose to purchase the service from National Statistics have received a weekly report on deaths of patients – the Public Health Mortality File. The report is prepared within a few days of the reporting of deaths, and therefore in some cases the cause of death does not take account of information that is obtained at a later date, for example confidential information supplied by registrars. Thus, the file is not appropriate as the basis for accurate statistics about causes of deaths, but can be used by Health Authorities to identify deaths certified as due to notifiable diseases and for calculating summary statistics about numbers of deaths. The file includes the name of the doctor certifying death, and the Health Authority was able to undertake a comparison of deaths of West Pennine residents certified by Shipman and those certified by other general practitioners, for the period late 1996 to June 1998. Using the data presented by the Authority, the death rate among women aged 65 or more in West Pennine was 2.7 per 100, but for Shipman the rate was 26.0 per 100.

The Authority also undertook an analysis using the family health services database (the Exeter System) of removals of patients from Shipman's registered list due to deaths. The patient registration component of the Exeter System contains the general identity details of patients registered with NHS general practitioners. It is linked electroncially with the National Health Service Central Register (NHSCR), and provides the base to calculate capitation payments to general practitioners and for the management of national screening programmes. In addition to recording details of when and with which practitioner each patient is registered, it contains details of patients removed from practitioners' lists and the reasons for removal, including death.

In this analysis, the Authority used a download from the Exeter System that included the dates of admission and removal from general practitioners' lists. The Authority considered that some deaths may not have been coded appropriately, and the numbers of deaths may therefore be an underestimate, although deaths occurring in hospital would have been included. An increasing number of deaths among women aged 65 or above was identified. In addition, 66.7% of Shipman's patients died in their own homes, but the proportion for all deaths in West Pennine was 19.2%.

The Authority undertook a third and more detailed analysis of mortality data provided by National Statistics and population data from the Exeter database. The death rates in Tameside and Glossop were used to calculate an expected death rate with which to compare the rate observed among Shipman's patients. For patients aged 65 and over (including males and females), rates of death among Shipman's patients were higher than expected for all years from 1993 to 1998. They were either as expected, or below the expected rate for 1990 to 1992, but above the expected rate between 1987 and 1989. No data were available before 1987. The total number of deaths in excess of the expected number among females aged 65 and over was 85 between 1993 and 1998.

## 2.4 The investigation by *Todmorden News and Advertiser*

A local investigation into the numbers of deaths during Shipman's appointment as a general practitioner in Todmorden has been undertaken by Peter Devine, the chief reporter of the local newspaper. The data were identified from the columns of the newspaper. The figures indicated an increase in the total numbers of deaths in the area during Shipman's appointment, with 401 deaths between 1st March 1974 and 30th September 1975. In the previous 19 months (1st August 1972 – 28th February 1974) there were 348 deaths, and in the 19 months following Shipman's departure there were 372. The number of death certificates signed by Shipman whilst working in Todmorden was identified as 22.

## 2.5 A preliminary review of deaths of Shipman's patients 1974–1998

### Background

The Births and Deaths Registration Act (1968) requires that in the case of the death of a person who was attended during the last illness by a registered medical practitioner, that practitioner shall sign a medical certificate of cause of death (MCCD) stating the cause of death, and shall deliver the certificate to the registrar. In addition to cause of death, the certificate should also state the deceased's name, age, and date and place of death.

The death must be notified to the registrar of the district in which the death took place by an informant, who is usually a relative of the deceased, or the person in charge of the institution in which the person died. The informant must provide details about the date and place of death, the full name and sex of the deceased, maiden name of married women, date and place of birth, and occupation and usual address. The data from the doctor's certificate and the informant are recorded in the register, and if the Registrar is satisfied that the death does not need to be reported to the coroner, a death certificate will be issued giving authority for burial or to apply for cremation.

The data recorded by registrars are collated by National Statistics to produce reports on national, regional and district death rates and causes of deaths. From 1993, a new computer database has been used at the Titchfield branch of National Statistics which includes all the data recorded by the registrar supplemented by automatic coding of causes of deaths in International Classification of Diseases (ICD9) format. This database may be searched for text terms, for example the name of the doctor signing the MCCD. Copies of the registrar's certificate of deaths (form 310(Rev)) are available for earlier years, and are stored as part of the National Deaths Register held at Southport. These forms can be searched to identify the doctor who issued the certificate.

### Method

In the audit, the following details from the information notified to National Statistics were of interest:

- General practitioner signing the MCCD

- Patient's name, age, sex

- Place of death

- Usual address

- Certified causes of death.

In order to judge whether the numbers of deaths certified by Shipman are in any way unusual, information about the numbers that would have been expected is required. In this preliminary analysis, deaths certified by a small number of general practitioners from the same locality were included. The criteria used to select the comparison local practitioners were: full-time practitioners, and in practice in the locality for all or most of the years during which Shipman was in practice. Six practitioners from Hyde and three from Todmorden met these criteria. All the Todmorden doctors, including Shipman, worked in the same practice. Since a part-time practitioner also worked in the practice and the practice had a shared list system, the part-timer was included in the comparison group.

National Statistics were asked to identify and provide copies of the death notifications of the patients of these practitioners, for the years 1977-98 for Hyde, and 1973-6 for Todmorden. Deaths prior to 1993 were identified by hand searches in Southport of files of death notifications from the relevant districts, Tameside in the case of Hyde and Calderdale in the case of Todmorden. Deaths from 1993 onwards were identified through searches of the computer database at Titchfield. In both searches, the key variable used to identify cases was the name of the practitioner signing the certificate. Some cases may have been overlooked in the searches. For example, the name of the practitioner may have been recorded inaccurately or illegibly.

Furthermore, hand searches of large numbers of records are laborious. To check for missing cases, the cremation registers at crematoria in the districts concerned were also reviewed (see Section Five).

## Findings

A total of 1657 MCCDs were identified as issued during the years of interest by the included general practitioners. 1555 were directly identified by National Statistics, and a further 102 were identified from cremation registers. These had not been identified by National Statistics because either the deaths had been registered in districts other than Tameside or Calderdale, (24 deaths were registered in Stockport, one patient of Shipman and 23 patients of the comparison practitioners), the name of the general practitioner had been recorded inaccurately (for example, Shipley rather than Shipman), or the death had been overlooked during hand searching.

Nine of the 102 cases identified through cremation registers had been certified by Shipman, and all these related to his period in Hyde. Of the comparison general practitioners in Todmorden for the years 1973–6, one additional case was identified for one practitioner, and two cases each for two other practitioners. Of the comparison practitioners in Hyde for the period 1977–98, the numbers of additional cases per general practitioner were 6, 10, 12, 18, 18 and 24.

It is likely that some other deaths have not been identified, in particular those followed by burials. Seventy-two percent of the 1657 deaths were followed by cremation and 102 were identified solely through cremation registers. If it is assumed that the proportion who were cremated was the same among the deaths identified by National Statistics and those not so identified, then it is probable that approximately 40 deaths followed by burials have not been included. This is only 2.4% of the total number of deaths, and can have no effect on the conclusions of the audit. It is also highly unlikely that the general practitioners would have issued more than one or two MCCDs for deaths registered in distant districts and that would not, therefore, have been identified in the audit. Furthermore, there is no reason why a particular general practitioner should have had an unusual number of such cases. Consequently, it can be concluded that virtually all MCCDs issued by the general practitioners were identified.

The findings are summarised in Tables 2.1 and 2.2. The place of death is categorised into home or institution, with institutions being either residential or nursing homes, or hospitals and hospices. A general practitioner may issue a MCCD in the case of a death in hospital if the practitioner has been attending the person during the last illness, and death occurs shortly after hospital admission. General practitioners may also issue certificates for deaths in community hospitals when they are attending the patient. A small number of deaths occurred in doctors' surgeries, and these have been included in the Tables as deaths 'at home'.

**Table 2.1. Numbers of deaths certified by Shipman and six comparison general practitioners, Hyde 1977–1998.**
(Deaths at home include deaths in doctors' surgeries; deaths in institutions include deaths in residential and nursing homes, hospitals and hospices).

| GP | Place | 77 | 78 | 79 | 80 | 81 | 82 | 83 | 84 | 85 | 86 | 87 | 88 | 89 | 90 | 91 | 92 | 93 | 94 | 95 | 96 | 97 | 98 | |
|---|---|---|---|---|---|---|---|---|---|---|---|---|---|---|---|---|---|---|---|---|---|---|---|---|
| Shipman | Home | 3 | 20 | 20 | 14 | 14 | 14 | 8 | 23 | 23 | 13 | 13 | 16 | 15 | 7 | 8 | 3 | 21 | 13 | 34 | 36 | 39 | 21 | 400 |
| | Inst | 1 | 8 | 9 | 8 | 12 | 7 | 7 | 8 | 3 | 2 | 5 | 4 | 2 | 2 | 4 | 4 | 8 | 4 | 5 | 7 | 8 | 3 | 121 |
| | Total | 4 | 28 | 29 | 22 | 26 | 21 | 15 | 31 | 26 | 15 | 18 | 20 | 17 | 9 | 12 | 7 | 29 | 17 | 39 | 43 | 47 | 24 | 521 |
| 1 | Home | 9 | 16 | 12 | 7 | 10 | 11 | 13 | 8 | 12 | 7 | 10 | 5 | 1 | 1 | 2 | 7 | 5 | 5 | 1 | | | | |
| | Inst | | 3 | 1 | 2 | 3 | 1 | 3 | 3 | 4 | 1 | 4 | 3 | 1 | 2 | 3 | 5 | 5 | 2 | 3 | 2 | | | |
| | Total | 9 | 19 | 13 | 9 | 13 | 12 | 16 | 11 | 16 | 8 | 14 | 8 | 2 | 3 | 5 | 12 | 10 | 7 | 4 | 2 | | | |
| 2 | Home | 8 | 9 | 8 | 10 | 8 | 10 | 8 | 10 | 6 | 6 | 3 | 10 | 8 | 8 | 12 | 3 | 2 | 2 | 1 | 6 | 3 | | |
| | Inst | 4 | 3 | 5 | 5 | 1 | 1 | 8 | 3 | 5 | 1 | 2 | 3 | | 2 | 1 | 6 | 3 | 5 | 4 | 3 | 2 | 2 | |
| | Total | 12 | 12 | 13 | 15 | 9 | 11 | 16 | 13 | 11 | 7 | 5 | 13 | 8 | 10 | 13 | 9 | 5 | 7 | 5 | 9 | 5 | 2 | |
| 3 | Home | 11 | 8 | 9 | 8 | 13 | 8 | 7 | 7 | 4 | 5 | 6 | 7 | 4 | 4 | | 5 | 1 | 3 | 1 | | 1 | | |
| | Inst | | 2 | 1 | 1 | 1 | 1 | 4 | | 1 | 1 | 3 | | 3 | | | 1 | 6 | 6 | 1 | | | | |
| | Total | 11 | 10 | 10 | 9 | 14 | 9 | 11 | 7 | 5 | 6 | 9 | 7 | 7 | 4 | | 6 | 7 | 9 | 2 | | 1 | | |
| 4 | Home | | | | | | | 5 | 11 | 6 | 4 | 7 | 3 | 7 | 4 | 2 | 3 | 3 | 5 | 5 | 1 | 1 | 1 | |
| | Inst | | | | | | | 4 | 8 | 5 | 4 | 2 | 7 | 3 | 1 | 7 | 3 | 3 | 5 | 3 | 4 | 6 | 2 | |
| | Total | | | | | | | 9 | 19 | 11 | 8 | 9 | 10 | 10 | 5 | 9 | 6 | 6 | 10 | 8 | 5 | 7 | 3 | |
| 5 | Home | 7 | 8 | 13 | 7 | 5 | 5 | 6 | 6 | 4 | 8 | 6 | 5 | 9 | 5 | 3 | 6 | 2 | 7 | 5 | 6 | 5 | 3 | |
| | Inst | 2 | 1 | 2 | 1 | | 3 | 4 | 3 | 1 | 1 | 2 | | 2 | 3 | 4 | 1 | 4 | 3 | 1 | 3 | 1 | 1 | |
| | Total | 9 | 9 | 15 | 8 | 5 | 8 | 10 | 9 | 5 | 9 | 8 | 5 | 11 | 8 | 7 | 7 | 6 | 10 | 6 | 9 | 6 | 4 | |
| 6 | Home | | | | | | 2 | 4 | 5 | 2 | 9 | 5 | 3 | 3 | | 1 | 4 | 3 | 4 | 2 | 2 | | 2 | |
| | Inst | | | | | | | 2 | 1 | 4 | 4 | 5 | 1 | 3 | 2 | 2 | 2 | 8 | 1 | 2 | 6 | 5 | | |
| | Total | | | | | | 2 | 6 | 6 | 6 | 13 | 10 | 4 | 6 | 2 | 3 | 6 | 11 | 5 | 4 | 8 | 5 | 2 | |

**Table 2.2. Numbers of deaths certified by Shipman and four comparison general practitioners, Todmorden 1973–1976.**
(There were no deaths in doctors' surgeries; deaths in institutions include deaths in residential and nursing homes, hospitals and hospices).

| GP | Place | 73 | 74 | 75 | 76 |
|---|---|---|---|---|---|
| Shipman | Home | | 3 | 16 | |
| | Inst | | 2 | 1 | |
| | Total | | 5 | 17 | |
| 1 | Home | 8 | 10 | 10 | 10 |
| | Inst | 3 | | 1 | 1 |
| | Total | 11 | 10 | 11 | 11 |
| 2 | Home | 16 | 13 | 15 | 11 |
| | Inst | 1 | 2 | 5 | 2 |
| | Total | 17 | 15 | 20 | 13 |
| 3 | Home | 3 | 3 | 6 | 7 |
| | Inst | 1 | | | 1 |
| | Total | 4 | 3 | 6 | 8 |
| 4 | Home | 11 | 6 | 12 | 9 |
| | Inst | | 3 | 1 | 5 |
| | Total | 11 | 9 | 13 | 14 |

There was a difference between Shipman and the comparison Hyde practitioners in the numbers of MCCDs they issued (see Table 2.1). Between 1977 and 1998, Shipman issued 499 MCCDs, 372 for deaths at home, six for deaths in the practice, and 121 for deaths in institutions. The total numbers issued by doctors 2, 3 and 5 in Hyde, who were working for almost the same period as Shipman, were 210, 145 and 178 respectively. There were eight deaths in doctors' surgeries, six being certified by Shipman, the other two being certified by two different general practitioners. Shipman's rate of issue of death certificates at Todmorden is comparable with other practitioners.

## Conclusions

In relation to the comparison practitioners, there was a high number of deaths among Shipman's patients. In Hyde, he issued MCCDs for 499 of his patients, but over the same period the next highest number of MCCDs issued by an individual practitioner was only 210, a difference of 289. There are potential explanations other than murder for the observed excess deaths, for example, the numbers of patients registered with each general practitioner, or characteristics of the patient population such as age, social class, or disease severity. The Tables also indicate considerable variation in the numbers of deaths certified by a general practitioner from year to year. Therefore, chance may be another potential explanation. Furthermore, the deaths included in the Tables are only those certified by general practitioners; deaths certified by hospital doctors or coroners are excluded. It should also be noted that on initial inspection, the number of MCCDs issued by Shipman when working in Todmorden is similar to other local practitioners (Table 2.2).

Thus, in order to draw conclusions about the patterns of deaths, it is necessary to supplement the evidence from death notifications with other evidence about the clinical practice of Harold Shipman.

The sources of evidence fall into four groups:

- numbers and characteristics of the patients registered with Shipman

- documentation of the clinical management of deceased patients, obtained from clinical records and cremation forms

- records of cases referred to the coroner

- death notifications of all patients registered with Shipman, irrespective of who signed the MCCD.

These sources of evidence are discussed in the following Sections.

# Three: Characteristics of patients registered with Harold Shipman

## 3.1 Numbers of patients

### Hyde

### Background

Most of the doctors of the group practice in which Shipman worked 1977–1991 operated as more or less independent practitioners with their own lists of patients. Shipman worked in this way, and therefore did not have a shared patient list.

According to Mr Justice Forbes' summing up of the trial, Shipman had told the court that his registered list of patients when he joined the practice in Hyde in 1977 was just over 2,000, but it grew to nearer 3,000 in the following years. He had reported that the list was a representative cross-section of the general population in terms of age and gender. Shipman also told the court that his list size was about 2,300 when he started practising as a single handed practitioner in 1992, that it increased to 3,200 which he found too much, and that he reduced it to 3,100.

### Method

It has not been possible to obtain independent information about the numbers of patients registered with Shipman between 1977 and 1987, but West Pennine Health Authority were able to provide details from 1987 onwards.

### Findings

Table 3.1 outlines the total numbers of patients in three age groups registered with Shipman and the comparison practitioners in Hyde on the first of October annually between 1987 and 1998. The Health Authority was also able to provide information about the numbers of males and females from 1991. His total list size was 2853 in 1987 and 3046 in 1998, reaching a peak of 3124 in 1994. In October of the year in which he became a single handed practitioner (1992), he had 2931 registered patients.

**Table 3.1. The numbers of patients registered with Shipman and the comparison practitioners, 1987–1998.**

| | 1987 | 1988 | 1989 | 1990 | 1991 | 1992 | 1993 | 1994 | 1995 | 1996 | 1997 | 1998 |
|---|---|---|---|---|---|---|---|---|---|---|---|---|
| **Shipman** | | | | | | | | | | | | |
| Females <65 | | | | | 1240 | 1280 | 1375 | 1360 | 1341 | 1329 | 1329 | 1345 |
| males <65 | | | | | 1215 | 1254 | 1340 | 1368 | 1353 | 1340 | 1339 | 1348 |
| *Total <65* | *2447* | *2448* | *2454* | *2471* | *2455* | *2534* | *2715* | *2728* | *2694* | *2669* | *2668* | *2693* |
| Females 65–74 | | | | | 115 | 127 | 131 | 134 | 120 | 122 | 120 | 113 |
| males 65–74 | | | | | 92 | 97 | 107 | 97 | 87 | 89 | 86 | 99 |
| *Total 65–74* | *218* | *219* | *227* | *209* | *207* | *224* | *238* | *231* | *207* | *211* | *206* | *212* |
| Females 75 + | | | | | 116 | 110 | 102 | 101 | 105 | 94 | 87 | 77 |
| males 75 + | | | | | 64 | 63 | 60 | 64 | 64 | 64 | 67 | 64 |
| *Total 65-74* | *188* | *188* | *182* | *180* | *180* | *173* | *162* | *165* | *169* | *158* | *154* | *141* |
| **Total list size** | **2853** | **2855** | **2863** | **2860** | **2842** | **2931** | **3115** | **3124** | **3070** | **3038** | **3028** | **3046** |
| | | | | | | | | | | | | |
| **1** | | | | | | | | | | | | |
| Females < 65 | | | | | 1237 | 1197 | 1177 | 1160 | 1123 | | | |
| Males < 65 | | | | | 1267 | 1253 | 1226 | 1216 | 1160 | | | |
| *Total < 65* | *2548* | *2545* | *2506* | *2457* | *2504* | *2450* | *2403* | *2376* | *2283* | | | |
| Females 65–74 | | | | | 191 | 192 | 194 | 186 | 172 | | | |
| Males 65–74 | | | | | 139 | 138 | 141 | 143 | 145 | | | |
| *Total 65–74* | *291* | *291* | *285* | *305* | *330* | *330* | *335* | *329* | *317* | | | |
| Females 75 + | | | | | 152 | 158 | 155 | 152 | 165 | | | |
| Males 75 + | | | | | 63 | 66 | 70 | 63 | 68 | | | |
| *Total 75+* | *217* | *199* | *202* | *187* | *215* | *224* | *225* | *215* | *233* | | | |
| **Total list size** | **3056** | **3035** | **2993** | **2949** | **3049** | **3004** | **2963** | **2920** | **2833** | | | |
| | | | | | | | | | | | | |
| **2** | | | | | | | | | | | | |
| Females < 65 | | | | | 1261 | 1246 | 1212 | 1191 | 1126 | 1093 | 1045 | 996 |
| Males < 65 | | | | | 1337 | 1324 | 1304 | 1266 | 1212 | 1181 | 1130 | 1060 |
| *Total< 65* | *1764* | *1782* | *2584* | *2513* | *2598* | *2570* | *2516* | *2457* | *2338* | *2274* | *2175* | *2056* |
| Females 65–74 | | | | | 143 | 136 | 142 | 137 | 136 | 125 | 119 | 116 |
| Males 65–74 | | | | | 107 | 95 | 97 | 104 | 104 | 105 | 98 | 72 |
| *Total 65–74* | *86* | *94* | *252* | *235* | *250* | *231* | *239* | *241* | *240* | *230* | *217* | *188* |
| Females 75 + | | | | | 120 | 117 | 109 | 110 | 111 | 122 | 126 | 132 |
| Males 75 + | | | | | 54 | 55 | 51 | 54 | 55 | 58 | 67 | 72 |
| *Total 75+* | *37* | *37* | *165* | *158* | *174* | *172* | *160* | *164* | *166* | *180* | *193* | *204* |
| **Total list size** | **1887** | **1913** | **3001** | **2906** | **3022** | **2973** | **2915** | **2862** | **2744** | **2684** | **2585** | **2448** |
| | | | | | | | | | | | | |
| **3** | | | | | | | | | | | | |
| Females < 65 | | | | | 1115 | 1091 | 1031 | 992 | | | | |
| Males < 65 | | | | | 1084 | 1025 | 997 | 979 | | | | |
| *Total < 65* | *2235* | *2220* | *2200* | *2162* | *2199* | *2116* | *2028* | *1971* | | | | |
| Females 65-74 | | | | | 121 | 118 | 116 | 114 | | | | |
| males 65-74 | | | | | 99 | 95 | 103 | 105 | | | | |
| *Total 65-74* | *242* | *239* | *229* | *224* | *220* | *213* | *219* | *219* | | | | |
| females 75 + | | | | | 119 | 112 | 116 | 117 | | | | |
| males 75 + | | | | | 51 | 53 | 50 | 51 | | | | |
| *Total 75+* | *158* | *157* | *163* | *163* | *170* | *165* | *166* | *168* | | | | |
| **Total list size** | **2635** | **2616** | **2592** | **2549** | **2589** | **2494** | **2413** | **2358** | | | | |
| | | | | | | | | | | | | |
| **4** | | | | | | | | | | | | |
| Females < 65 | | | | | 825 | 824 | 823 | 806 | 802 | 797 | 769 | 680 |
| Males < 65 | | | | | 948 | 946 | 950 | 949 | 936 | 933 | 917 | 905 |
| *Total <65* | *1719* | *1762* | *1761* | *1737* | *1773* | *1770* | *1773* | *1755* | *1738* | *1730* | *1686* | *1585* |
| Females 65-74 | | | | | 91 | 91 | 90 | 88 | 83 | 80 | 76 | 73 |
| Males 65-74 | | | | | 78 | 79 | 85 | 81 | 81 | 78 | 75 | 77 |
| *Total 65-74* | *181* | *176* | *168* | *161* | *169* | *170* | *175* | *169* | *164* | *158* | *151* | *150* |
| Females 75 + | | | | | 113 | 109 | 99 | 86 | 88 | 85 | 89 | 89 |
| Males 75 + | | | | | 60 | 60 | 56 | 56 | 59 | 55 | 54 | 50 |
| *Total 75+* | *158* | *157* | *167* | *172* | *173* | *160* | *155* | *142* | *147* | *140* | *143* | *139* |
| **Total list size** | **2058** | **2095** | **2096** | **2070** | **2115** | **2100** | **2103** | **2066** | **2049** | **2028** | **1980** | **1874** |

| Table 3.1. Continued. | | | | | | | | | | | |
|---|---|---|---|---|---|---|---|---|---|---|---|
| | **1987** | **1988** | **1989** | **1990** | **1991** | **1992** | **1993** | **1994** | **1995** | **1996** | **1997** | **1998** |
| **5** | | | | | | | | | | | | |
| Females < 65 | | | | | 1098 | 1090 | 1067 | 1036 | 1010 | 1002 | 977 | 972 |
| Males < 65 | | | | | 1120 | 1115 | 1096 | 1087 | 1073 | 1073 | 1034 | 1022 |
| *Total <65* | *2273* | *2237* | *2213* | *2193* | *2218* | *2205* | *2163* | *2123* | *2083* | *2075* | *2011* | *1994* |
| Females 65–74 | | | | | 149 | 150 | 155 | 160 | 150 | 146 | 148 | 133 |
| Males 65–74 | | | | | 114 | 113 | 109 | 115 | 103 | 99 | 103 | 99 |
| *Total 65–74* | *261* | *268* | *268* | *275* | *263* | *263* | *264* | *275* | *253* | *245* | *251* | *232* |
| Females 75 + | | | | | 121 | 119 | 118 | 116 | 115 | 121 | 123 | 134 |
| Males 75 + | | | | | 50 | 54 | 54 | 54 | 72 | 99 | 72 | 73 |
| *Total 75+* | *184* | *172* | *176* | *163* | *171* | *173* | *172* | *170* | *187* | *220* | *195* | *207* |
| **Total list size** | **2718** | **2677** | **2657** | **2631** | **2652** | **2614** | **2599** | **2568** | **2523** | **2540** | **2457** | **2433** |
| | | | | | | | | | | | | |
| **6** | | | | | | | | | | | | |
| Females < 65 | | | | | 1077 | 1031 | 958 | 953 | 921 | 915 | 870 | 851 |
| Males < 65 | | | | | 1171 | 1109 | 1073 | 1057 | 1032 | 998 | 959 | 938 |
| *Total < 65* | *1607* | *1568* | *1717* | *1479* | *2248* | *2140* | *2031* | *2010* | *1953* | *1913* | *1829* | *1789* |
| Females 65–74 | | | | | 173 | 172 | 171 | 171 | 170 | 161 | 150 | 141 |
| Males 65–74 | | | | | 126 | 129 | 120 | 128 | 120 | 118 | 108 | 102 |
| *Total 65–74* | *259* | *239* | *239* | *246* | *299* | *301* | *291* | *299* | *290* | *279* | *258* | *243* |
| Females 75 + | | | | | 173 | 166 | 156 | 149 | 156 | 161 | 167 | 159 |
| Males 75 + | | | | | 99 | 95 | 96 | 91 | 93 | 79 | 84 | 79 |
| *Total 75+* | *199* | *208* | *213* | *213* | *272* | *261* | *252* | *240* | *249* | *240* | *251* | *238* |
| **Total list size** | **2065** | **2015** | **2169** | **1938** | **2819** | **2702** | **2574** | **2549** | **2492** | **2432** | **2338** | **2270** |

There are some differences between Shipman's list and those of the comparison practitioners, illustrated in Figures 3.1 and 3.2. In 1987, the percentage of patients aged 75 and above were similar, but in the following years, in Shipman's list the percentage declined. In contrast, in the majority of the comparison group the mean percentage increased, although there was a slight decline for doctor 4. The percentage of patients registered with Shipman aged 65–74 was lower than the comparison practitioners throughout the period 1987–1998. Table 3.1 indicates that the numbers of females aged 75 or above registered with Shipman declined between 1991 and 1998 from 116 to 77, although the numbers of males remained reasonably constant at about 64. It should be noted that in November 1997 Shipman's practice undertook an audit of patients who left the practice. The most common reason for leaving the practice (37.5% of those leaving) was moving to a new address served by a different Health Authority. The second most common reason for leaving the practice list was death (27.9% of those leaving the practice) (see Appendix 4).

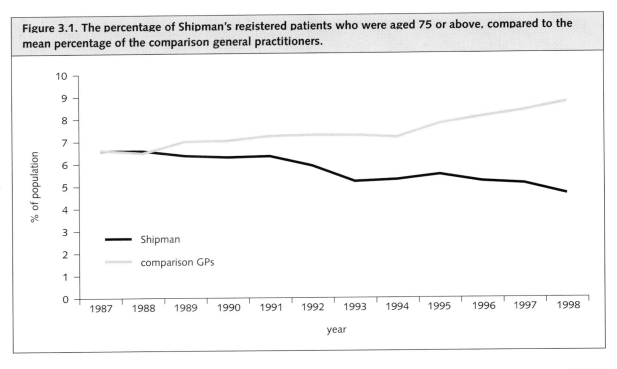

**Figure 3.1. The percentage of Shipman's registered patients who were aged 75 or above, compared to the mean percentage of the comparison general practitioners.**

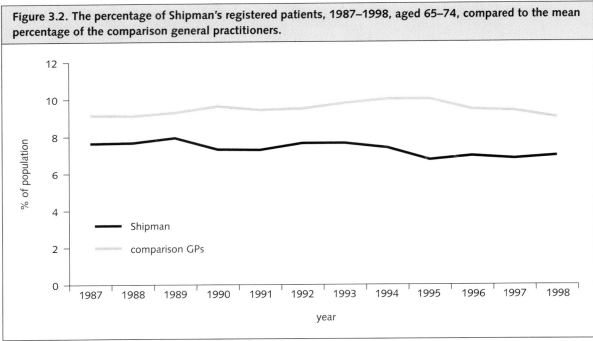

**Figure 3.2. The percentage of Shipman's registered patients, 1987–1998, aged 65–74, compared to the mean percentage of the comparison general practitioners.**

## Conclusions

Shipman had a relatively large list, which was greater than the average for full time unrestricted principals in general practice in England (2001 in 1992 and 2022 in 1998 (Statistical Bulletin, 2000)) and the list sizes of the comparison general practitioners, although most of them also had higher than the average numbers of patients (Table 3.1). Nevertheless, between 1987 and 1998 his list size was relatively stable.

In group practices, the numbers of patients registered with a general practitioner may not be an accurate indication of the number cared for by that practitioner. For example, a new partner in a practice may initially have no registered patients until new patients join the practice. However, the new partner will probably take an equal share of the work of consulting and visiting patients. There may also be relatively sudden changes in list size. For example, when a doctor leaves a practice, the remaining partners may decide to divide the list between them. Factors such as these are unlikely to have had a substantial impact on Shipman's list since the group practice in which he worked from 1977 – 1992 operated a policy in which the practitioner had direct responsibility for his or her own registered patients. However, some of the comparison practitioners probably operated shared list systems, and a shared list system was in operation in Todmorden in 1974 and 1975.

Since Shipman had a relatively high number of patients in Hyde, a proportionately high number of deaths would be expected. Thus, the total number of registered patients should be taken into account, although it should be noted that some of the comparison practitioners had similar numbers of patients (general practitioners 1 and 2). In contrast, Shipman had a lower proportion of patients aged 65–74 than the comparison practitioners, and a falling proportion aged 75 or above. Both these factors would normally be expected to be associated with a lower total number of deaths.

## Todmorden

Accurate information about the numbers of patients registered with the Todmorden practice is not available. The memory of a general practitioner who worked in the practice during the relevant years suggests that the list was at least 10,000, and could have been 12,000. The earliest accurate information relates to 1990, when the total number of registered patients was 14170 (11686 aged 0-64, 1368 65–74, and 1116 aged 75 or above).

The patient list in Todmorden was shared, and accurate information about the number of patients for whom Shipman was clinically responsible is not available. However, he was working full time and can be assumed to have been responsible for a commensurate share of all patients at the practice. If the list size is assumed to have been approximately 11,000 people, and the number of whole time equivalent general practitioners in the practice taken as 4.5, he would have a nominal list of 2,444.

# 3.2 Jarman Scores

The Jarman index is a measure of factors that increase demand on general practitioners' services (Jarman, 1985). The national average is set at 0, with positive values indicating above average demand and negative scores below average demand.

## Hyde

The Jarman scores were calculated from data provided by West Pennine Health Authority, including the numbers of patients of each practitioner resident in each electoral ward, and the Jarman scores for the wards. The scores for the practice lists as at October 1998 were relatively similar, Shipman's being 13.67, doctors 3, 4 and 5 being 13.43, doctor 2 being 13.93 and doctor 6 14.29. The scores indicate that the doctors in the audit all cared for patient populations likely to have a greater than average demand for care.

## Todmorden

The Jarman score for Todmorden was taken from data provided by Calderdale and Kirklees Health Authority. Todmorden is itself a discrete electoral ward, and most patients in the ward were assumed to be registered with the practice. The Jarman score for the ward is 17.1 and therefore this score was applied to the patients of all the Todmorden practitioners, including Shipman.

## Conclusions

There were only minor differences in Jarman scores between the patients of general practitioners in Hyde, and the same score applied to patients of the practitioners in Todmorden. Therefore, differences in Jarman scores are unlikely to explain differences in the mortality rates of the patients of Shipman and the comparison practitioners.

# 3.3 Townsend Scores

The Townsend score is also derived from indices identified in the 1991 census – unemployment, non-ownership of a car, non-ownership of a home and overcrowding. (Townsend et al, 1988). It measures relative material deprivation, the average score being set at 0, with positive numbers indicating above average deprivation and negative numbers lower than average deprivation.

## Hyde

The scores were calculated from Townsend scores for electoral wards and the number of patients of the included practices resident in each ward. For Shipman's practice, the score was 1.63, the score for general practitioners 3, 4 and 5 was 1.68, and for general practitioners 2 and 6 the scores were 1.85 and 1.93 respectively.

## Todmorden

The Townsend score for Todmorden is 0.66, and this was applied to all the patients of the practice.

# 3.4 Conclusion

There were only marginal differences in Townsend scores between the patients of Shipman and the comparison practitioners in Hyde. The Townsend score for Todmorden applied to the patients of both Shipman and the comparison practitioners. Therefore, differences in the levels of material deprivation are unlikely to explain any observed differences in mortality rates. Both Todmorden and Hyde had higher than average Jarman and Townsend scores, indicating a moderate degree of deprivation. The mortality rates in these districts would therefore be expected to be higher than the national average.

# Four: Review of Clinical Records of Deceased Patients

## 4.1 Introduction

A review of the clinical records of Shipman's deceased patients was undertaken (a) to identify cases sharing features found in the convictions, (b) to assess the relationship between the certified cause of death and the recorded medical history and (c) to review the integrity of the records.

General practitioners are required to keep adequate records of the illnesses and treatment of patients on forms supplied for that purpose, and the records must be returned to the local Health Authority if the patient dies. The guidance of the General Medical Council published in 1995 stated that doctors must "keep clear, accurate, and contemporaneous patient records which report the relevant clinical findings, the decisions made, information given to patients and any drugs or other treatment prescribed" (GMC, 1995).

The most commonly used general practice records are often referred to as "Lloyd George" records since their general format can be traced to, or before, Lloyd George's Insurance Act of 1911. Paragraph 36 (6) of the Terms of Service for General Practitioners (Statutory Instrument 635, 1992) requires that the doctor shall forward records to the Health Authority on request as soon as possible, and within 14 days of being informed by the Authority of the death of a person on his or her list, and in any other case of death, not later than one month of learning of such a death.

Prior to July 1994, Health Authorities were required to retain the records of deceased patients for a minimum of three years. However, this policy was replaced by an obligation to retain records for ten years after a patient's death (Department of Health, 1994). It was also advised that general practitioners should arrange secure storage of records used and retained within the surgery. The guidance was repeated in 1998 (Department of Health, 1998), with additional provisions in relation to records of service personnel. Both the 1994 and 1998 guidance advise that the views of the profession's local representatives be obtained on the need to retain records after the expiry of the minimum period.

However, it appears that some Health Authorities adopted a policy of offering to return records to the patients' general practitioner. General practitioners may choose to retain records for medico-legal reasons or for clinical audit of deaths. West Pennine Health Authority did operate such a policy, and Shipman did request the return of records. Thus, although some records of deceased patients were available from West Pennine Health Authority, the police had found others in Shipman's possession – either in a cardboard box in the garage at his home or in a plastic bag on the dresser in his house. This method of storing records is clearly not in accordance with the spirit of the guidance of HSC 1998/217 (Department of Health, 1998).

All the clinical records of cases reported to them by relatives or others had been collected and held as evidence to their inquiry by the Greater Manchester Police, who gave permission for their review. Fifteen records believed to be still preserved could not be traced or were not available for review. Therefore, a total of 231 were available, grouped by the Greater Manchester Police according to the weight of evidence identified to suggest murder (Table 4.1). The records included a group of 94 that had not been investigated by the police and remained unclassified. Fifty-one other records had been stored by the Health Authority and these were also reviewed.

**Table 4.1. The numbers of records reviewed in relation to classification of cases by the Greater Manchester Police.** An additional 51 records had been stored by the Health Authority, and therefore a total of 282 were reviewed.

| | Number of patients | Records preserved | Records available for review |
|---|---|---|---|
| Convictions | 15 | 15 | 15 |
| Sufficient evidence | 31 | 30 | 30 |
| Insufficient Evidence | 80 | 58 | 49 |
| No evidence | 63 | 49 | 43 |
| Other records held by the police | 94 | 94 | 94 |
| Total | 283 | 246 | 231 |

The review of records was undertaken in four stages:

- A review of the records of the 15 patients that Shipman was convicted of murdering (referred to subsequently as the convictions). This review was undertaken to establish the features typical of murder.

- A review of the remaining records of patients for whom Shipman issued MCCDs in order to establish the circumstances of death, including presence or absence of the typical features.

- A review of all 282 records to assess the quality of record keeping.

- A review of a sample of records to assess the integrity of recording. The audit trail of the computer records was employed in this review. Following Shipman's arrest, the police had taken a copy of the data held on his practice computer system, thus providing a complete duplicate of the records held on his computer as they were on 7th September 1998.

Each record consisted of the standard medical record envelope and its contents, including continuation cards completed by the attending practitioner, results of investigations ordered by the general practitioner, and copies of correspondence to and from specialists and hospitals. In addition, each record was supplemented by a comprehensive print out from the practice computer. Some records also included other information obtained by the police, for example a copy of the death notification, or items from hospital records. All this material was reviewed.

In giving evidence to the trial, Shipman reported that from 1992 he had used both computer and hand written medical records in the single handed practice. He said he used hand written records to detail particularly confidential information that he did not want the patient to see, arguing that it would have been possible for patients to see some computer entries during their consultations. He also claimed to use the Lloyd George cards to make notes when on home visits. However, information about visits would commonly be recorded on a standard form that was attached to the notes when a visit was made, the information from the form being transferred to the computer after completion of the visit. Almost certainly, these visit forms were destroyed once details had been entered into the computer, since few were found during the record review. Those that were found usually contained only the information noted by the practice receptionist at the time the request for the visit was made, and did not contain information recorded by Shipman.

To ensure the validity of inferences drawn from the records, dual independent review of samples of records was undertaken. Two experienced general practitioners were asked to review selected records, paying particular attention to the relationship between clinical history and certified cause of death. The reviewers did not have access to the findings of the record review undertaken by myself, (RB) and were asked to form their own views solely on the basis of the content of the records.

One practitioner reviewed the records of convicted cases and a sample of cases classified as 'no evidence', a total of 43 records. The second practitioner reviewed the cases classified as 'sufficient evidence' plus a sample classified as 'no evidence', a total of 38 records. Thus, a total of 81 comparisons between an independent reviewer and reviews by RB were available. The reviews were compared to identify differences in the history of the terminal illness and in the assessment of the relationship between certified cause of death and history.

There was a substantive difference in only one case, in which the independent reviewer failed to note that the coroner had been contacted to discuss the death. In all other cases (98.8%), there were no differences about the clinical history. There were no major differences in views on the relationship between cause of death and recorded clinical history, but there were differences in ten cases (12.3%) in the level of concern expressed by the reviewers. In six cases, RB expressed a greater degree of concern about the relationship between recorded history and certified cause of death, and in four cases the independent reviewer expressed greater concern.

# 4.2 The convictions

## Background

The clinical records of the convictions were reviewed first. These cases had been the subject of detailed investigation by the police and searching review during the trial. In consequence, the true circumstances leading to death had been determined. The review of these records was supplemented by additional evidence presented at the trial. Therefore, it was possible to identify from these cases those features typical of murder. In the subsequent review of the records of other patients, evidence to indicate the presence of absence of these features was sought.

## Methods

Each record was reviewed in order to identify and record the variables listed in Table 4.2. In order to protect the confidentiality of these patients, the findings relating to each case have not been included in this report. The details in the records were supplemented by the evidence presented at the trial, as summarised by the Honourable Mr Justice Forbes.

| Table 4.2. Information collected from the clinical records. |
|---|
| **Variable** |
| 1   Cause of death as recorded on record envelope |
| 2   Date of death |
| 3   Gender |
| 4   Place of death as indicated in the records |
| 5   Summary of key elements of past medical history |
| 6   Information recorded on continuation cards about the terminal illness |
| 7   Information recorded on the practice computer about the terminal illness |
| 8   Information about the terminal illness from other sources e.g. hospital summaries, letters from the ambulance service, notes from deputising doctors |
| 9   Findings from review of the computer audit trail |
| 10  Long term medication |
| 11  Aspects of cause of death diagnosed by Shipman |
| 12  Aspects of cause of death diagnosed by other doctors |
| 13  Assessment of relationship between certified cause of death and history recorded in the records |
| 14  Adequacy of information recorded about time and place of death, persons present, treatment given and whether an ambulance had been called |
| 15  Discrepancies between manual and computer record entries |
| 16  Any other reasons for doubt about the integrity of the records |
| 17  Record of prescription of opiate medication |
| 18  Other observations on the records |

## Findings

The records of the murders for which Shipman was convicted reveal a distinct set of features:

- The victims were all older females (age range 49-82 years; eleven were aged over 65).

- Shipman was present at the death, or recorded as seeing the patient shortly before death. In five cases Shipman's records indicated that he was present at the death. In the other cases, the records indicated that he had seen the patient the day before death or earlier on the day of death, even a few minutes before death.

- Sudden death at home, often in the afternoon. Fourteen deaths were reported as occurring between 13.30 and 18.15 and one at approximately 10.00 hours.

- A weak association between the cause of death and clinical history. The records may have indicated the presence of an illness, but usually did not suggest that the illness was sufficiently severe as to threaten life. During the trial, witnesses gave evidence that the victims had not appeared to be seriously ill in the period before their deaths.

- In many cases, a referral to the coroner would have been normal or required practice, but Shipman had usually told relatives that a post mortem would not be necessary.

- In at least three cases, Shipman made no attempt to resuscitate patients who died in his presence.

- In at least three cases, Shipman claimed that he had telephoned to summon an ambulance, but when the patient had died he had cancelled the ambulance. However, itemised telephone billing records indicated that no calls from the patients' homes had been made to Greater Manchester Ambulance Service.

- Seven records were altered by Shipman before and/or after the patient's death in order to fabricate a history relevant to the certified cause of death.

- False entries were made on two cremation forms about the people present at the moment of death and the period during which Shipman had attended the patient during the final illness. During the trial, Shipman claimed that these entries were errors, and it was agreed by counsel for the defence that his record keeping was poor.

- The causes of death given by Shipman were commonly heart conditions (8) or cerebrovascular disease (3). He also gave pneumonia (2), cancer (1) and old age (1) as causes of death.

- Nine victims had been buried. In each of these cases, toxicological investigations led the Home Office Pathologist to determine that the cause of death had been morphine toxicity.

A number of general points about the records can also be made. They were characterised by their brevity, the legibility of the writing on the continuation cards was often poor, and the use of duplicate records systems (paper and computer) led to a confused account of patient care.

## Conclusions

A set of features typical of the murders of which Shipman was convicted has been identified. The clinical records of other deceased patients could be expected to contain information to enable detection of some of these features. These include whether Shipman recorded being present at the death or attending the patient shortly before death, the place of death, the age and gender of the patient, and the cause of death and its relationship to the clinical history contained in the records. It should also be noted that Shipman's records were poor and that he had been shown to have made back-dated, false entries.

# 4.3 The records of other patients for whom Shipman had issued MCCDs

## Background

The records of these patients were reviewed to determine the circumstances of death, and to identify cases that demonstrated the features typical of the convictions.

## Methods

Of the 282 records available, 15 were the convicted cases and were excluded. Of the remainder, 87 occurred in hospital and these were also excluded. Thus, 180 cases were included in this assessment of the circumstances of death.

The information collected from the records is listed in Table 4.2. Since Shipman made liberal use of abbreviations, a glossary is provided in Table 4.3. In the extracts from the records, Shipman's punctuation has generally been followed.

Following the collection of data from the records, each case was classified according to the level of suspicion about the cause of death. Level of suspicion was rated as either low, moderate or high, and determined by the extent to which cases exhibited the features typical of the murders of which Shipman was convicted:

- whether Shipman was present at the death,

- whether Shipman was present shortly before the death,

- sudden deaths at home

- the relationship between the certified cause of death and clinical history.

Table 4.3. Glossary of abbreviations used by Shipman in his clinical records (abbreviations appear in both upper and lower case in the records).

| Abbreviation | Explanation |
| --- | --- |
| a/e | Air entry |
| Bp | Blood pressure |
| Bs | Blood sugar |
| Cert | Medical certificate of cause of death (MCCD) |
| Chf | Congestive heart failure |
| c/o | Complaining of |
| Ct | Coronary thrombosis |
| Cva | Cerebrovascular accident (i.e. stroke) |
| D | Diagnosis |
| Dc | Death certificate (MCCD) |
| Dm | Diabetes mellitus |
| Esr | erythrocyte sedimentation rate |
| Hb | Haemoglobin |
| HS | Heart sounds |
| IHD | Ischaemic heart disease |
| Jvp | Jugular venous pressure |
| L | Left |
| lvf | Left ventricular failure |
| nos | Not otherwise specified |
| OA | Osteoarthiritis |
| O/E | On examination |
| qds | Four times daily |
| R | Right |
| ra | Rheumatoid arthritis |
| Re | With reference to |
| Rx | Treatment |
| S/hill | Stepping Hill Hospital |
| si jt | Sacroiliac joint |
| tluk | 'to let us know' |
| 2fb | Two finger's breadth |
| UTI | Urinary tract infection |
| v | Visit |

The certified cause of death was used to indicate the suddenness of death. Thus, deaths due to heart problems or strokes were assumed to be sudden, unless otherwise indicated in the records. Deaths primarily due to cancer were regarded as not sudden, unless the records indicated otherwise. A proportion of deaths were classified as due to old age, the cause of death being given as old age, senility, dementia or even 'natural causes'. It was assumed that deaths in this category were gradual unless details given in the records indicated otherwise.

The relationship between certified cause of death and history was judged in two ways. First, the details given by Shipman were used, and a judgement made as to whether they were typical of the normal clinical course of illness. Second, the records were reviewed for evidence of external validation of the certified cause of death by a health professional other than Shipman. For example, the diagnosis of terminal cancer by a hospital specialist or the confirmation of a severe stroke by a locum or deputising doctor would serve to validate deaths certified as due to these conditions. Thus, the classification of cases into different levels of suspicion depended to some extent on clinical judgement used to interpret the information contained in the records.

Information about the integrity of records is presented later. Evidence about the falsification of records did not play a major role in the audit in judging the level of suspicion about the circumstances of death. This information was available for only a small proportion of records – those with computer records. The audit trail system was installed on Shipman's Microdoc computer system from 14th October 1996. Therefore, no evidence is available about alterations or additions to computer records prior to that date. It was not possible to reliably judge whether paper records had been altered.

# Findings

Table 4.4 shows the proportions of cases showing the typical features for which Shipman was convicted. Accordingly, 38 (21.1%) of the 180 cases were classified as not suspicious, 39 (21.7%) as moderately suspicious, and 102 (56.7) as highly suspicious. The level of suspicion could not be determined for one case because very little information was contained in the record, and this case has been excluded from the results that follow.

**Table 4.4. Numbers of cases classified as not suspicious, or moderately or highly suspicious, showing those displaying features typical of the cases for which Shipman was convicted. N=179 (in one case, the level of suspicion could not be determined).**

| Level of suspicion | | None | Moderate | High |
|---|---|---|---|---|
| Present at death | Yes | 0 | 3 | 27 |
| | No | 30 | 25 | 68 |
| | Not clear | 8 | 11 | 7 |
| Seen within 1 day of death | Yes | 13 | 8 | 48 |
| | No | 17 | 19 | 52 |
| | Not clear | 8 | 12 | 2 |
| Cause relates to Shipman's history | Good | 16 | 3 | 0 |
| | Some | 13 | 16 | 41 |
| | No | 5 | 9 | 56 |
| | Not clear | 4 | 11 | 5 |
| Evidence from another doctor to support certified cause of death | Yes | 26 | 11 | 6 |
| | No | 7 | 17 | 91 |
| | Not clear | 5 | 11 | 5 |
| Place of death | Home | 14 | 29 | 97 |
| | Practice | 0 | 0 | 4 |
| | Nursing home | 9 | 3 | 0 |
| | Residential home | 15 | 7 | 1 |
| Cause of death | Cardiac | 5 | 19 | 52 |
| | CVA | 7 | 6 | 27 |
| | Cancer | 13 | 6 | 1 |
| | Old age etc | 8 | 5 | 12 |
| | Other | 5 | 3 | 10 |

The mean age of those classified as not suspicious was 78 years, moderately suspicious 77 years and highly suspicious 78 years. The gender of patients according to level of suspicion about the cause of death is shown in Table 4.5. Of the 126 deaths among females, 81(64.3%) were classified as highly suspicious. Of the 53 deaths among males, 21 (39.6%) were classified as highly suspicious. The median age of women in the highly suspicious group was lower than in the moderately or not suspicious groups (Table 4.6).

**Table 4.5. Gender of patients in cases classified as highly, moderately or not suspicious. N=179.**

| Level of suspicion | None n (%) | | Moderate n (%) | | High n (%) | |
|---|---|---|---|---|---|---|
| Male | 16 | (42.1) | 16 | (41.0) | 21 | (20.6) |
| Female | 22 | (57.9) | 23 | (59.0) | 81 | (79.4) |
| Total | 38 | (100.00) | 39 | (100.00) | 102 | (100.00) |

**Table 4.6. Median age (interquartile range, minimum, maximum) of male and female patients for whom Shipman issued MCCDs, classified into highly, moderately or not suspicious following review of surviving clinical records. (n=179).**

| Level of suspicion | Males | | | | Females | | | |
|---|---|---|---|---|---|---|---|---|
| | median | inter-quartile range | min | max | median | inter-quartile range | min | max |
| None | 72.6 | 27.9 | 38.2 | 91.6 | 87.5 | 13.6 | 63.0 | 97.8 |
| Moderate | 73.2 | 19.9 | 43.2 | 89.0 | 82.0 | 11.7 | 11.7 | 104.7 |
| High | 81.0 | 13.4 | 64.2 | 90.4 | 77.0 | 8.8 | 53.1 | 89.2 |

Deaths classified as highly suspicious were more likely to have occurred on Mondays and Tuesdays, and less likely to occur to occur on Saturdays and Sundays (Table 4.7).

**Table 4.7. Numbers of deaths on different days of the week in groups classified as either highly, moderately or not suspicious. N=179.**

| Level of suspicion | Monday | Tuesday | Wednesday | Thursday | Friday | Saturday | Sunday | Total |
|---|---|---|---|---|---|---|---|---|
| | N (%) | N (%) | N (%) | N (%) | N (%) | N (%) | N (%) | |
| None | 5 (15.6) | 7 (20.0) | 4 (14.3) | 7 (21.2) | 7 (25.9) | 6 (46.2) | 2 (18.2) | 38 |
| Moderate | 6 (18.8) | 7 (20.8) | 6 (21.4) | 9 (27.3) | 7 (25.9) | 2 (15.3) | 2 (18.2) | 39 |
| High | 21 (65.6) | 21 (60.0) | 18 (64.3) | 17 (51.5) | 13 (48.1) | 5 (38.5) | 7 (63.6) | 102 |
| Total | 32 (100) | 35 (100) | 28 (100) | 33 (100) | 27 (100) | 13 (100) | 11 (100) | 179 |

In the case of sudden death, the cause was frequently certified by Shipman as either a cerebrovascular accident or heart condition (coronary thrombosis, ischaemic heart disease, left ventricular failure, congestive heart failure). In many of the deaths certified as due to a cerebrovascular accident, death took place unusually quickly. Typically, Shipman records attending the patient within one day of death and finding vague symptoms or signs. In such circumstances, he frequently indicates a 'watch and wait' management plan by using the letters 'tluk' – to let us know if the condition deteriorates. Case 537 is a typical example (each case is referred to in the audit by a unique code number).

> Case 537. Computer record: *day before death* – h/o vertigo. Falls to r 150/100 r leg ? weak ? plantar left all ok stemetil sachets tluk if alters. *day of death* – o/e – dead. Neighbour saw at 1400 ok found 1500 in bed dead cva bp.

Shipman's records of deaths certified as due to heart conditions were often similar, the patient being seen shortly before death with relatively mild symptoms, then being found dead within a few hours or the next day. Some records also indicated that the doctor was present at death. Case 502 is an example, certified as a coronary thrombosis.

> Case 388: Continuation card: *date of death* – visit c/o pain in chest HS I II 40/m a/e = normal; no sign failure 90/40 pain on off all night like indigestion D – CT, CHF IV 10mg morphine patient (illegible) died 13.30.

Case 388 also illustrates another feature giving rise to concern. In many cases of sudden death at which he was present, he did not call for help or attempt resuscitation. In this case, the general practitioner had time to take a history, examine the patient and administer pain relief, but did not have time to summon an ambulance. The normal course of action when confronted by a seriously ill patient would be to immediately summon help.

Sudden death could also be ascribed to other causes, as in case 431.

> Case 431: Computer record: *date of death* – Seen in own home. influenza with bronchopneumonia; noisy chest wishes to stay at home, amox *date of death* found dead, amb present.

Old age could also be given as the cause of sudden death, (case 488), or even 'natural causes', for example case 443.

> Case 488: continuation card: *date of death* – 1415 found unconscious. Not unwell felt tired. Old age. No other illness. Computer record: *date of death* – O/E – dead old age.

> Case 443: continuation card: 10 *days before death* visit. OK *day of death* visit. Found dead + 2000hr *day after death* – DC natural causes (old age) police and home help present.

Nineteen records indicated that opiates had been prescribed, and in eight cases this was in the course of terminal care. One patient received pethidine tablets. Seven received intravenous morphine (10mg) and two intravenous diamorphine (10mg) for acute myocardial infarction or heart failure (for example, see case 388). The British National Formulary recommends slow intravenous injection (2mg/minute) of 10mg morphine in acute myocardial infarction or acute pulmonary oedema, followed by a further 5–10mg if necessary, with doses reduced by half in frail or elderly people. The recommended doses for diamorphine are half those for morphine. Thus, Shipman was recording administration of these drugs at the upper limit of the recommended dose range.

In addition to the features identified from the convictions, the review of the additional 180 records pointed to another feature that could give rise to suspicion. In eighteen cases, the records indicated that the patient had allegedly refused hospital admission, with Shipman consequently planning to revisit the patient later the same day or the next day. Patients were either reported as found dead later by a relative, neighbour or carer, or found dead by Shipman when he returned. Case 520 is a typical example.

> Case 520: Computer record: *date of death* – c/o a pain. Chest hips all night heavy type pain breathless a little tired no energy ? sweaty hips oa o/e pulse 66 hs I II bp 100/60 nausea probable ct needs admission not happy revisit *date of death* – o/e – dead. GM ambulance service

In a small number of other cases, Shipman records calling for an ambulance, but then cancelling the call when the patient collapsed and died. In such circumstances, an attending general practitioner would usually attempt resuscitation until the ambulance arrived. The convictions included cases in which Shipman claimed to have called for, but subsequently cancelled, an ambulance, but in these cases no telephone record of the calls could be found.

> Case 161: Continuation card: *date of death* – v history of being ill from Sat (2/7) vague chest pain tingling L arm breathless sweaty felt faint – looks ill pulse 60/m BP 90/? Basal creps D – probably CT with myocardial failure given 10mg morphine IV neighbour (illegible) ambulance (illegible) cancelled patient died approx 2.00 self & neighbour present undertaker informed/(illegible) DC CT, chronic bronchitis emphysema.

## Conclusions

Of the 179 records that contained sufficient information to enable a judgement to be formed about the level of suspicion in relation to the circumstances of death, 102 (56.7%) were classified as highly suspicious. A further 39 (21.7%) were classified as moderately suspicious. The classification rests on clinical judgement based on interpretations of clinical records and was unable to take into account evidence from other sources such as relatives or friends of patients. It is likely, therefore, that some of the deaths classified as suspicious may have been entirely natural.

Nevertheless, it is clear that the cases classified as highly or moderately suspicious did share many of the features typical of the convictions. Most died at home, and had either been seen within one day of death or with Shipman present at death. The clinical histories given by Shipman often did not relate convincingly to the certified cause of death and evidence to corroborate the cause of death from other doctors was frequently not available. Although females formed the majority of patients in the highly suspicious group, the deaths of 21 males were also classified as highly suspicious. On the basis of the review of surviving records, there is, therefore, considerable reason for concern about the cause of death of substantially more patients than those of which Shipman was convicted.

# 4.4 Quality of recording

## Background

During the trial. Shipman claimed to have made errors in his record keeping, and it was admitted by the counsel for the defence that his record keeping was poor. A review of the deceased patients' records was therefore undertaken to determine the quality of Shipman's records.

## Methods

All 282 deaths with records available were included in this review. Information was collected about two aspects of recording – the general condition of the records and recording in relation to patient management. The information collected is shown in Table 4.8.

| Table 4.8. Information collected to assess quality of records | |
| --- | --- |
| 1 | Whether the records were arranged in date order |
| 2 | Whether there was a summary of the patient's history in the records |
| 3 | Whether the records were legible |
| 4 | Adequacy of information recorded about the principal complaint, management given, prescribing |
| 5 | Whether the records indicated that chronic diseases were managed systematically |

The general condition of the records was judged by whether they were arranged in date order, whether there was a completed summary, and the legibility of the writing. The information about patient management assessed in the review included adequacy of recording of prescribing, information about the presenting complaint and patient management, and evidence of systematic management of chronic disorders such as hypertension, diabetes or Parkinson's disease.

## Findings

It was unusual for Shipman's records to be arranged in date order (Table 4.9). This may be partly explained by the repeated reviews of these records during the police investigation. However, the records that had not been reviewed previously were also not in order. In contrast, 250 (88.7%) records had a completed summary card, even when the computer record was the preferred record system. In general, the summary cards were up to date.

| Table 4.9. The number (%) of records that were arranged in date order, (N=282). | | |
|---|---|---|
| Arranged | n | % |
| no | 266 | 94.3 |
| yes | 13 | 4.6 |
| unclear | 3 | 1.1 |

The handwriting on the continuation cards was poor (Table 4.10). Sometimes the writing was completely illegible, even though the clinical details related to serious symptoms or deaths. Shipman's records also tended to be brief or even perfunctory (Tables 4.11-13). The contrast between Shipman's entries and some locums was marked – the locums recorded more details and their writing was usually more legible.

| Table 4.10. The number (%) of records judged to be legible. 'Not applicable' applies to records that did not contain any writing by Shipman. (N=282). | | |
|---|---|---|
| Legibility | n | % |
| poor | 30 | 10.6 |
| variable | 228 | 80.9 |
| uniformly adequate | 19 | 6.7 |
| not applicable | 5 | 1.8 |

| Table 4.11. The quality of information recorded about prescribing. (N=282). | | |
|---|---|---|
| Rating of prescribing information | n | % |
| very little recorded | 43 | 15.2 |
| incomplete information recorded | 113 | 40.1 |
| complete information recorded | 75 | 26.6 |
| not receiving prescriptions | 42 | 14.9 |
| unclear | 9 | 3.2 |

The recording of information about prescribing was frequently poor (Table 4.11). Those prescriptions issued using the computer prescribing system were appropriately and adequately recorded on the computer. However, information about prescriptions issued during home visits or on other occasions when the computer was not used was usually incomplete. Most commonly, the amount prescribed was not recorded, but other details were occasionally omitted or the writing was illegible. Prescriptions for controlled drugs such as diamorphine must be written by hand and not printed by computer, and information about the prescribing of these drugs was generally poor. Almost invariably, Shipman failed to record the batch numbers of medication he personally gave by injection. On reviewing the controlled drugs registers in local pharmacies (see Section Seven) it was evident that large numbers of prescriptions had been issued to a few patients during terminal care. However, the recording of their medication was often incomplete; for example, in one case (484) only a fraction of the medication dispensed was noted in the records to have been administered to the patient.

| Table 4.12. The quality of information recorded about presenting complaints (N=282). In some records, the presenting complaint could not be determined, and it was not possible to judge the completeness of recording. | | |
|---|---|---|
| Adequacy of information about presenting complaints | n | % |
| little or no information | 100 | 35.5 |
| some information, but incomplete | 155 | 55.0 |
| adequate information | 16 | 5.7 |
| good | 1 | 0.4 |
| not possible to judge | 10 | 3.5 |

| Table 4.13. Adequacy of information about patient management in relation to the terminal illness or most recent episode of care. 'Not clear' indicates cases in which no care had been provided by Shipman in the recent past. (N=282). | | |
|---|---|---|
| Information about patient management | n | % |
| none | 91 | 32.3 |
| very little | 155 | 55.0 |
| moderate | 23 | 8.2 |
| complete | 5 | 1.8 |
| not clear | 8 | 2.8 |

The information Shipman recorded about patient's clinical complaints was usually brief, both in paper or computer records. Cases 434 and 487 are typical examples:

> Case 434: Continuation card: *date* V chest tight A/E= BS (illegible). Further antibiotics ceporex (illegible).

> Case 487: Computer record: *date* cerebro arteriosclerosis dizzy start aspirin 75.

His recording of information about the circumstances of death was also commonly remarkably brief, for example cases 381 and 460.

> Case 381: Continuation card: *Date* amoxil 250mg sore throat (illegible) ok.
> *date* – (10 days later) + old age cerebro arteriosclerosis.

> Case 460: Computer records: *date* chronic obstructive airways disease. Chest better.
> *date* (1 day later) seen in own home O/E – dead. Old age.

In some cases, the recording of information about the management of chronic diseases such as hypertension or diabetes was good. This generally applied to records made by the practice nurse during routine long term patient management. Some records included disease specific chronic disease management record cards, and the computer records also demonstrated cases of appropriate systematic management.

However, when patients were managed solely by Shipman, the records reflected his usual approach, with brief entries and poor handwriting (Table 4.14).

| Table 4.14. Evidence in the records to indicate systematic management of chronic disease. 'Not applicable' relates to patients with no chronic disease (N=282). | | |
| --- | --- | --- |
| Systematic management of chronic disease | n | % |
| nil or poor | 34 | 12.1 |
| moderate | 96 | 34.0 |
| good | 90 | 31.9 |
| not applicable | 62 | 22.0 |

## Conclusions

Shipman clearly took care to complete a summary for each patient that contained key details of the clinical history. His staff were also careful to record information about the routine management of chronic disorders, when they had a role in this task. Apart from these points, Shipman's record keeping was consistently poor.

His writing was sometimes illegible, but of greater concern was the lack of detail he recorded about patients' presenting complaints and his clinical management. This problem was exacerbated by the use of dual record systems – paper and computer. Entries in either system were usually brief, and on many occasions consultations were recorded on only one system. Relatively few practices report using only computer notes during consultations (Waring, 2000), and although Shipman appears to have recorded the majority of his consultations on the practice computer from 1994 onwards, his policy on when to record entries in the computer or paper systems (or both) was unclear. Furthermore, although information about prescriptions was adequate when the computer was used, handwritten information about prescriptions was usually poor. The quantity of medication issued was often omitted, and the batch numbers of injected drugs were not recorded.

It can be argued, therefore, that Shipman's record keeping was not in compliance with the Terms of Service for general practitioners or GMC guidance. This conclusion rests on a review of a relatively large sample of records, but it is likely that a review of a small sample, such as might be incorporated into regular appraisals or revalidation, would have disclosed the problem of poor recording. Furthermore, the findings should prompt concern about the extent to which a combination of an out moded paper recording system and the variable use of computer records impairs the quality of the records of other general practitioners.

# 4.5 Integrity of records

## Background

Integrity of records is defined by the Joint Computing Group as "the property that data have not been altered or destroyed in an unauthorised manner" (Joint Computing Group, 2000). Evidence was presented at the trial that Shipman had made back-dated entries in computer records, and Shipman generally argued that these entries were made to record the clinical history given to him by patients shortly before they died. Since, he claimed, they told him of symptoms they experienced up to several months before, he dated the entries to match the histories they had given him. However, the entries in question generally read as if they were written at the time rather than days or months after they actually occurred; some even included findings of clinical examinations such as blood pressure. In explaining one such instance, he claimed that it was an error. Shipman also had a habit of entering information about home visits that took place in the afternoon on the following morning. During the trial, Shipman claimed that he was aware of the audit trail feature of his Microdoc computer system and that he knew how to deceive the audit trail by changing the internal date of the computer. He reported that he had been the chairman of the local user group of the company that had supplied the computer system, and was a member of the national user group. The audit trail facility had been discussed in detail at one or more of the user group meetings.

Requirements for accreditation (RFA) of general practice computer systems were introduced in 1993. The RFA specifies a core set of requirements that all general practice computer systems should be capable of performing. The fourth version of the RFA was published in June 1997 and included mandatory requirements relating to security and confidentiality. A revised RFA was published in 1999. Microdoc is RFA version 4 compliant, but is not yet registered under RFA (99). RFA version 4 stipulates that systems should require user passwords and have an audit trail that holds information about any changes made to the records (General medical practice computer systems RFAV4, 1997). The information must include the identity of the user (determined by the password), and the date and time of the transaction. The system should allow the practitioner to view the audit trail.

## Methods

The copy of Shipman's computer system taken by the police following his arrest on 7th September 1998 was used. The audit trail had been installed on 14th October 1996, and could be accessed from the recorded entry for each consultation by one or two key strokes. It indicated the date and time the entry had been made, derived from the computer's own internal date and time. Thus, the computer trail makes it possible to detect entries made on dates different to the dates indicated by the person using the computer. The computer also notes the person making the entry, determined by the password used to access the system by the computer user.

The computer records of the convictions and those cases classified by the Greater Manchester Police as either having sufficient evidence or no evidence for gaining convictions were reviewed. As there was no computer record for 12 of these, information was available for 59. The cases for which no records were available included those of patients who had died before Shipman had installed or begun to use his computer system, or those in which he had made no computer entries.

## Findings

Of the 59 records, evidence of entries made after the indicated date were found in seven. Two of these were convictions, two cases classified as having sufficient evidence for conviction, and three in cases classified as having no evidence. The convictions will not be considered further. Of the other cases, the falsified entries appear to have been made to indicate a history appropriate to the certified cause of death. For example, in case 565 in which death was certified as due to coronary thrombosis, additional entries were made after death to suggest a history of transient ischaemic attacks. In case 556, an entry was made the day before death to indicate a consultation three days before death at which the blood pressure was checked. The death was certified as due to a stroke. In case 560, an entry was made on the day of death to indicate a consultation the day before at which an extending stroke had been diagnosed. In case 568, an entry had been made three hours after death to indicate a consultation one week before at which the patient's hypertension had been reviewed. The cause of death was certified as a stroke.

In four other cases, entries were made the day after death to record the circumstances of death. Typically, these entries were made by Shipman between 8.30 and 8.45 am. For example, in case 517, an entry for a visit to the patient on the previous morning was made, recording a history typical of myocardial infarction. A second entry was made to record the death as taking place the same afternoon.

## Conclusions

In several of the convictions, evidence was presented to suggest that Shipman had made entries in paper records to fabricate a relevant clinical history. For example, in one case dates of entries had been checked with the known whereabouts of the patient to show that the consultation had not taken place on the date suggested by Shipman. In the audit it was not possible to obtain external verification of recorded consultations or other evidence to raise questions about the veracity of entries in the paper records or computer entries made before October 1996. In consequence, a comprehensive assessment of the extent to which Shipman created false entries in his records has not been possible. The findings that are available do confirm that falsely dated entries were made relating to consultations that may or may not have taken place, but suggest that this did not occur frequently. It was an occasional feature of the murders for which Shipman was convicted, or of cases that can be regarded as suspicious.

In coming to a conclusion about the integrity of the records, other factors should also be taken into account. An assessment of the extent to which the cause of death given by Shipman relates to details recorded in the records has already been presented (see Table 4.4). Of the 179 deaths that occurred under Shipman's care either in the patient's home, in the practice, or in a residential or nursing home, there was no discernible relationship between the cause of death and the history recorded by Shipman in 70 (39.1%). In an additional 70 (39.1%) cases, the relationship was only partly established. In 20 (11.2%) there was insufficient information available to form a judgement, and in only 19 (10.6%) was there a clear association. Furthermore, only 43 (24.0%) records contained information from another doctor such as a locum or hospital specialist that gave a history consistent with the certified cause of death. In addition, Shipman's recording habits were far from adequate. The use of two recording systems created confusion about patient management. Some patient contacts were recorded on paper only, others on the computer only, and others on both. On other occasions there were long breaks in recording, even though the patient had a chronic illness and was receiving medication, making it likely that some consultations had not been recorded at all.

The confusion was aggravated by the nature of Shipman's record entries. His recording of patient history, examination and management was economical at best, and frequently brief or even perfunctory. Details of prescriptions issued were often incomplete, unless issued through the computer system. The computer records were particularly short. The paper records were also marred by poor legibility. Partly as a consequence of the superficial record entries, it is difficult in many cases to clearly identify the justification for working diagnoses, or the reasons for management decisions.

A further problem of Shipman's recording system was the failure to retain, or perhaps even make, contemporaneous notes. This applies in particular to recording information about visits to patients. The visit form may or may not have been used by Shipman to record information that was subsequently transferred to the computer. Since the majority of visit forms have not been retained, it is impossible to judge the completeness of information recorded during visits and whether full details were indeed transferred to the computer. Several steps were required to ensure information about visits was recorded in the computer and Shipman was able to suggest during the trial that innocent errors were the cause of inaccurate record entries.

Nevertheless, it would be reasonable to speculate that Shipman's recording inaccuracies and irregularities could in some instances have been systematic attempts to conceal criminal acts. A review of a small sample of records of Shipman's deceased patients undertaken without knowledge of the evidence presented to the trial would probably lead to the judgement that the practitioner was over confident and possibly incompetent. An investigation of the audit trail would have been required to reveal the true circumstances.

A further point deserves consideration. The National Health Service Regulations require that practitioners return records to the Health Authority if a patient dies or on request of the Health Authority. In the case of computer records, a copy may be sent in written form or, with the consent of the Authority, in another form. However, in common with other general practice computer systems, Shipman's computer does not permit the deletion of records of patients who have died or left the practice. This is compatible with RFA version 4. The Data Protection Commissioner has accepted that until electronic records can be reliably transferred between practices, or between a practice and a Health Authority, an interim arrangement is required. Records of patients who have left the practice should be rendered inactive or archived, and not normally accessible in the system unless a valid reason for access arises. Wherever an inactive record is accessed, a record of the reason must be kept (Joint Computing Group, 2000). Since a steadily increasing number of records of deceased patients or patients who have left the practice are being retained on general practice computer systems, computer system suppliers should be encouraged to expedite the introduction of archiving arrangements.

# 4.6 Conclusions of the review of clinical records

It was possible to identify from the convictions a set of seven features associated to varying degrees with murder:

- all were older females

- Shipman was present at or shortly before death

- death often occurred at home in the afternoon

- the association between certified cause of death and clinical history was weak

- several patient records had false entries

- some cremation forms had false entries

- the stated causes of death were most commonly stroke or heart conditions, although cancer, pneumonia and old age were also stated.

The first three features were relatively strongly associated with the convictions, and the remaining four less strongly associated.

The review of the available records of those other patients for whom Shipman had issued MCCDs disclosed many cases in which some of these features could be identified (Table 4.4). Shipman had recorded being present at the death of 30 patients, had attended 69 within one day of death, and given heart conditions as the cause of death in 76. In 140 cases, death had occurred at the patient's home. A clear relationship between the clinical history recorded by Shipman and the certified cause of death was identified in only 19 cases, and evidence from a doctor other than Shipman that indicated a history relevant to the cause of death was identified in 43 cases. Consequently, of the total of 179 cases, 102 were classified as highly suspicious, and 39 as moderately suspicious. Since the level of suspicion was determined on the basis of the clinical records, it is not a definitive assessment of the true cause of death in any particular case. Additional evidence such as that identified by the police and presented at the trial would be needed to establish whether an individual had been murdered. Nevertheless, in three of the 102 highly suspicious cases, coroner's inquests have concluded that the patients were killed unlawfully, and inquests are to be held into a further 21 cases.

It is also clear that the quality of Shipman's record keeping was poor. Indeed, in some instances his use of dual record systems and brief record entries could reasonably be regarded as a deliberate ploy to conceal illegal activities. Nevertheless, it has proved impossible to judge the extent to which he fabricated entries in his paper records, or his computer records prior to October 1996, but this possibility should be kept in mind when interpreting the findings from his clinical records. He also fabricated entries on cremation forms.

# Five: Cremation forms

## 5.1 Background

The regulations governing cremation are laid down in the Statutory Rules and Orders, 1930, made under section 7 of the Cremation Act 1902 and section 10 of the Births and Deaths Registration Act, 1926. The Rules and Orders currently in force are those as amended by the cremation (Amendments) Regulations, 2000. The Regulations govern the maintenance and inspection of crematoria and the certification procedures that must be followed. Various forms are used at different stages of the required process to gain authority for cremation from the medical referee.

In outline, the forms used in virtually all deaths certified by general practitioners are Forms A to D. Form A is the application from the executor or nearest relative for the cremation to take place. Form B is completed by the medical practitioner who has attended the deceased during the last illness and can certify definitely as to the cause of death. Form C is a confirmatory medical certificate that is completed by another medical practitioner who has been qualified for not less than five years, and is not a relative of the deceased or a relative or partner of the doctor who has completed Form B. Form D gives authority for cremation, and is completed by the medical referee.

Crematorium staff are required to record each cremation in a register (otherwise referred to as 'Form G'). Forms A-D must be retained for a period of fifteen years, but the cremation register must be retained indefinitely. The Statutory Rules and Orders empower the Secretary of State, the Minister of Health or the Chief Officer of any police force to appoint someone to inspect cremation registers and documents. The authority of the Secretary of State was granted to inspect relevant records held at specific crematoria for the purposes of the audit.

## 5.2 Methods

Information was collected from the documents held by crematoria relating to the deaths of patients of Shipman and the comparison group of general practitioners. The cremation register at each crematorium was reviewed to identify all cremations since 1973 for which the practitioners had completed Form B. All available Forms B and C were reviewed, and all the crematoria serving the districts in which Shipman worked were included. These were Dukinfield and Stockport crematoria for Hyde and Burnley, Elland and Rochdale for Todmorden. The total numbers of cremations in 1996 and 1997 in each of these crematoria are shown in Table 5.1.

| Table 5.1. The annual number of cremations at the included crematoria, 1996 and 1997. | | |
|---|---|---|
| Crematorium | 1996 | 1997 |
| *Hyde* | | |
| Dukinfield | 2,308 | 2,240 |
| Stockport | 2,452 | 2,501 |
| | | |
| *Todmorden* | | |
| Burnley | 1,738 | 1,929 |
| Elland | 1,832 | 1,977 |
| Rochdale | 1,550 | 1,476 |

A copy of the Form B and Form C used at Dukinfield crematorium is included in Appendix 2. The information collected from each form is shown in Table 5.2.

| Table 5.2. Information collected from the cremation forms. |
| --- |
| **Information collected** |
| **Form B** |
| 1   Date and time of death |
| 2   Place of death |
| 3   GP a relative of the deceased or has a pecuniary interest |
| 4   How long the GP had attended the patient |
| 5   How long the GP had attended the patient in the last illness |
| 6   When the GP last saw the patient alive |
| 7   Examination of the patient after death |
| 8   Cause of death |
| 9   Mode and duration of death, and basis for these observations |
| 10   Individuals providing nursing during the last illness |
| 11   Persons present at death |
| 12   Any reasons for doubt about the cause of death |
| |
| **Form C** |
| 1   The practitioner has seen and examined the deceased |
| 2   The practitioner has questioned the attending doctor |
| 3   The practitioner has questioned any other person |

# 5.3 Findings

## Form B

The proportion of deaths followed by cremation has been gradually increasing, from 55% in 1970, to 65% in 1980, to 72% in 1997 (Cremation Society of Great Britain, 1999). Of the 1,657 deaths included in the audit from 1973 to 1998, 1192 (72%) were followed by cremation, with 65% of deaths in the 1970s and 74% of deaths in the 1990s being followed by cremation. Of the 521 deaths certified by Shipman, 390 (75%) were followed by cremation. The total number of deaths certified by all the comparison general practitioners combined was 1136, of which 802 (71%) were cremated.

A total of 767 cremation forms were still available for review, 64% of the 1192 cremations. 292 were patients of Shipman, and 475 patients of the comparison practitioners. In all but five cases, the general practitioner completing Form B had also issued the medical certificate of cause of death. The were no differences in the median age of cremated patients between general practitioners (Table 5.3). A higher proportion of Shipman's patients were female, 69.9% in comparison with 54.1% for the comparison practitioners (Tables 5.4 and 5.5), a trend that was consistent throughout 1985–1998, other than in 1985 and 1995.

| Table 5.3. The mean age (and 95% confidence intervals) of cremated patients of Shipman and the comparison practitioners. | | |
| --- | --- | --- |
| GP | Median (yrs) | Interquartile range |
| Shipman | 79.0 | 11.0 |
| 1 | 75.5 | 19.5 |
| 2 | 78.0 | 17.00 |
| 3 | 77.0 | 16.5 |
| 4 | 82.0 | 14.00 |
| 5 | 80.0 | 15.8 |
| 6 | 81.0 | 15.0 |

**Table 5.4. The numbers and % of patients of each general practitioner who were female ($X_6^2 = 23.9$; $p - 0.001$).**

| GP | Number of females | % female |
|---|---|---|
| Shipman | 204 | 69.9 |
| 1 | 46 | 53.5 |
| 2 | 44 | 44.9 |
| 3 | 34 | 56.7 |
| 4 | 44 | 55.0 |
| 5 | 49 | 58.3 |
| 6 | 40 | 59.7 |

Although crematoria are required to retain cremation forms for fifteen years, some forms were available from 1979. However, the preservation of these early records was inconsistent and an increasing proportion of cremation forms from 1984 or earlier were missing (Table 5.5). Since only relatively small numbers of forms for 1979–1984 were available, information about these years should be treated with caution.

If the findings are related to the years of patients' deaths, it is possible to identify the extent to which the key features found in the convictions can be detected in past years. Table 5.5 presents information about the numbers of females in each year from 1980 to 1998.

Some sections of occasional cremation forms had not been completed, and therefore the figures in the tables that follow do not always reach the totals of 292 for Shipman and 475 for the comparison practitioners.

**Table 5.5. Numbers of patients of Shipman and comparison practitioners who were cremated each year, 1979–1998, and the cremation forms were still available. The Table also shows the number and % of females. No patients of Shipman were cremated in 1992.**

| year | Shipman | | | Comparison GPs | | |
|---|---|---|---|---|---|---|
| | Total | Females | % female | Total | Females | % female |
| 1979 | | | | 2 | 1 | 50.0 |
| 1980 | 8 | 4 | 50.0 | 10 | 4 | 40.0 |
| 1981 | 6 | 4 | 66.7 | 6 | 4 | 66.7 |
| 1982 | 10 | 8 | 80.0 | 22 | 7 | 31.8 |
| 1983 | 5 | 2 | 40.0 | 10 | 4 | 40.0 |
| 1984 | 2 | 2 | 100.0 | 3 | 2 | 66.7 |
| 1985 | 18 | 12 | 66.7 | 44 | 31 | 70.5 |
| 1986 | 15 | 10 | 66.7 | 36 | 22 | 61.1 |
| 1987 | 14 | 10 | 71.4 | 45 | 23 | 51.1 |
| 1988 | 20 | 14 | 70.0 | 48 | 27 | 56.3 |
| 1989 | 21 | 14 | 66.7 | 43 | 18 | 41.9 |
| 1990 | 4 | 3 | 75.0 | 26 | 17 | 65.4 |
| 1991 | 2 | 1 | 50.0 | 21 | 10 | 47.6 |
| 1992 | – | | | 26 | 13 | 50.0 |
| 1993 | 23 | 16 | 69.6 | 35 | 23 | 65.7 |
| 1994 | 15 | 10 | 66.7 | 36 | 15 | 41.7 |
| 1995 | 33 | 19 | 57.6 | 18 | 13 | 72.2 |
| 1996 | 36 | 25 | 69.4 | 19 | 10 | 52.6 |
| 1997 | 41 | 33 | 80.5 | 20 | 11 | 55.0 |
| 1998 | 19 | 17 | 89.5 | 5 | 2 | 40.0 |
| total | 292 | 204 | 69.9 | 475 | 257 | 54.1 |

**Table 5.6. Place of death of patients of Shipman and the comparison practitioners.**
($X_5^2 = 36.8$; $p - 0.000$).

|  | Shipman | | Comparison GPs | |
| --- | --- | --- | --- | --- |
|  | N | % | N | % |
| home | 226 | 77.4 | 294 | 61.9 |
| residential home | 36 | 12.3 | 122 | 25.7 |
| nursing home | 24 | 8.2 | 40 | 8.4 |
| hospital | 0 |  | 15 | 3.2 |
| practice | 5 | 1.7 | 1 | 0.2 |
| other | 1 | 0.3 | 3 | 0.6 |
| total | 292 | | 475 | |

Table 5.6 shows that higher proportions of Shipman's patients compared to other practitioners died at home (77.4% v 61.9%) and on the practice premises (1.7% v 0.2%).

Figure 5.1 shows that from 1984, the proportion of deaths at home among Shipman's patients exceeded the proportion among the comparison practitioners. The details relating to 1979-84 must be regarded with caution.

There was also a difference between Shipman and the comparison practitioners in hour of death. 55% of his patients were reported by Shipman as dying between 13.00 and 19.00 but the proportion for the comparison doctors was 25%. The distribution of recorded hour of death is shown in Figure 5.2.

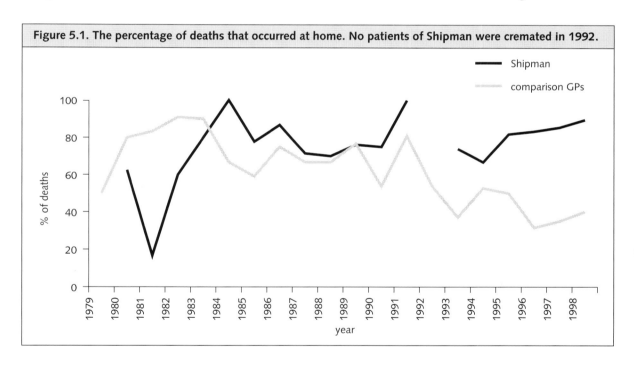

**Figure 5.1. The percentage of deaths that occurred at home. No patients of Shipman were cremated in 1992.**

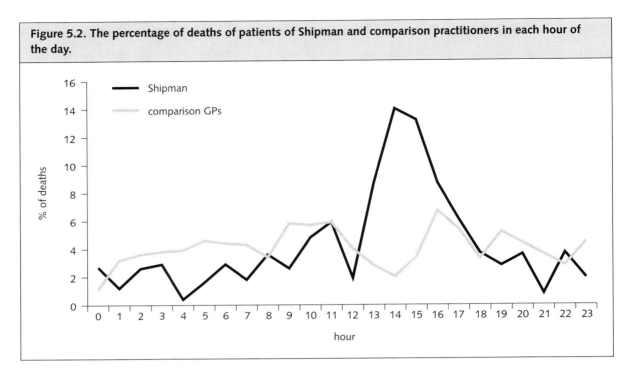

**Figure 5.2. The percentage of deaths of patients of Shipman and comparison practitioners in each hour of the day.**

**Table 5.7. Certified causes of death grouped into five categories, for MCCDs issued by Shipman and the comparison practitioners.** ($X^2_4 = 86.6$; $p - 0.000$).

|  | Shipman | | Comparison GPs | |
|---|---|---|---|---|
|  | N | % | N | % |
| cardiac | 102 | 34.9 | 123 | 25.9 |
| cerebrovascular | 61 | 20.9 | 38 | 8.0 |
| cancer | 45 | 15.4 | 159 | 33.5 |
| old age | 44 | 15.1 | 24 | 5.1 |
| other | 40 | 13.7 | 131 | 27.6 |
| total | 292 |  | 475 |  |

In relation to certified cause of death (Table 5.7), Shipman was more likely than the other practitioners to give cardiac conditions (myocardial infarction, ischaemic heart disease, heart failure), cerebrovascular accidents and old age as causes of death, but less likely to state cancer or other causes. Shipman certified 55.8% of deaths as due to either cardiac problems or stroke compared to 33.9% by other practitioners. Figure 5.3 shows that the proportion of deaths certified by Shipman as due to strokes or cardiac problems in each year exceeded the proportion for the comparison practitioners in most of the years 1980–1998.

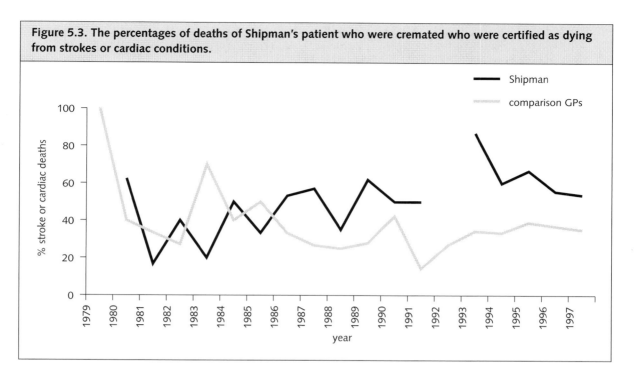

**Figure 5.3. The percentages of deaths of Shipman's patient who were cremated who were certified as dying from strokes or cardiac conditions.**

There were no meaningful differences between Shipman and the comparison practitioners in the number of weeks they reported attending patients in the last illness. Information recorded by the practitioners indicated that they chose different events as indicating the start of an illness, and any observed differences were due to inconsistent recording habits. The interval between last attending the patient and death is less open to interpretation, and in Shipman's case the interval was shorter than that of the other practitioners. The mean for Shipman was 49 hours, but for the other practitioners combined it was 88 hours, a difference of 39 hours (95% confidence interval 23 – 56 hours). Among Shipman's patients, there were no differences in the mean number of hours between male and female patients, or among those aged above or below 65.

**Table 5.8. Administrative information recorded on Form B by Shipman and comparison practitioners.**

|  | Shipman | | Comparison GPs | | |
|---|---|---|---|---|---|
|  | N | % | N | % | P |
| not a relative of the deceased | 292 | 100 | 472 | 99.4 | Ns |
| no pecuniary interest | 292 | 100 | 475 | 100 | Ns |
| ordinary attendant of the deceased | 290 | 99.3 | 456 | 96.2 | 0.01 |
| no doubt about the cause of death | 292 | 100 | 475 | 100 | Ns |
| not due to violence, poison or neglect | 291 | 99.7 | 473 | 99.6 | Ns |
| no reason for further examination | 291 | 99.7 | 474 | 99.8 | Ns |
| issued certificate | 292 | 100 | 463 | 97.5 | Ns |

There were no differences between Shipman and the comparison practitioners in the recording of background details – being a relative of the deceased, whether the practitioner had a pecuniary interest in the case, whether the practitioner attended the patient during the last illness or had doubts about the cause of death, and whether the practitioner has issued the MCCD (Table 5.8). Shipman was marginally more likely to report being the ordinary medical attendant of the deceased, a finding likely to be explained by his status as a single-handed practitioner from 1992 onwards.

Table 5.9 indicates that Shipman was present at death in 19.5% of instances compared to 0.8% amongst his colleagues, and that relatives or carers were present at only 40.1% of deaths of Shipman's patients compared to 80.2% for his fellow practitioners. There were also differences in the clinical aspects recorded, including the speed at which death took place (Table 5.10), and the recorded mode of death

(Table 5.11). 60.4% of his patients were reported by Shipman as dying within 30 minutes (Table 5.10). The equivalent percentage for the comparison practitioners was 22.7%.

Figure 5.4 shows that the percentage of Shipman's patients dying within 30 minutes was relatively high during most years 1980–1998. Shipman reported being present at death when this occurred in a residential or nursing home on only two occasions (3% of the total number of deaths of his patients in such accommodation). The equivalent number for the comparison general practitioners was also 2 (1% of deaths in residential or nursing homes).

**Table 5.9. The numbers of cases in which Shipman or the comparison practitioners reported being present at the death.** ($X_2^2 = 154.5$; $p - 0.000$).

|  | Shipman | | Comparison GPs | |
|---|---|---|---|---|
|  | N | % | N | % |
| no one | 118 | 40.4 | 90 | 19.0 |
| general practitioner | 57 | 19.5 | 4 | 0.8 |
| relatives or carers | 117 | 40.1 | 380 | 80.2 |
| total | 292 | | 474 | |

**Table 5.10. Length of time over which death occurred as recorded by Shipman and the comparison practitioners.** ($X_7^2 = 13.5$; $p - 0.000$).

|  | Shipman | | Comparison GPs | |
|---|---|---|---|---|
|  | N | % | N | % |
| seconds only | 82 | 29.0 | 23 | 5.1 |
| less than 29 minutes | 89 | 31.4 | 79 | 17.6 |
| 30 mins – 2 hours | 10 | 3.5 | 40 | 8.9 |
| 2 – 24 hours | 66 | 23.3 | 153 | 34.2 |
| 1 – 3 days | 21 | 7.4 | 116 | 25.9 |
| 4 – 7 days | 11 | 3.9 | 23 | 5.1 |
| 8 days – 4 weeks | 4 | 1.4 | 10 | 2.2 |
| 4 weeks plus | 0 | | 4 | 0.9 |
| Total | 283 | | 448 | |

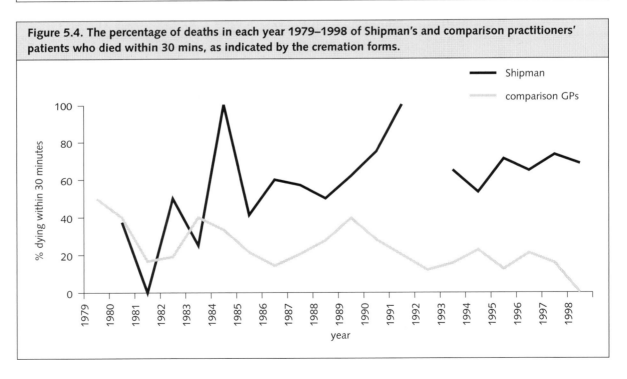

**Figure 5.4. The percentage of deaths in each year 1979–1998 of Shipman's and comparison practitioners' patients who died within 30 mins, as indicated by the cremation forms.**

| Table 5.11. Mode of dying recorded by Shipman and the comparison practitioners. ($X_6^2 = 127.2$; $p - 0.000$). | | | | |
|---|---|---|---|---|
| **Mode of dying** | **Shipman** | | **Comparison GPs** | |
| | N | % | N | % |
| syncope | 92 | 31.5 | 82 | 17.3 |
| collapse | 67 | 22.9 | 33 | 6.9 |
| coma | 121 | 41.4 | 221 | 46.5 |
| exhaustion | 3 | 1.0 | 106 | 22.3 |
| other – sudden | 1 | 0.3 | 17 | 3.6 |
| other – gradual | 3 | 1.0 | 15 | 3.2 |
| no details recorded | 5 | 1.7 | 1 | 0.2 |
| total | 292 | | 475 | |

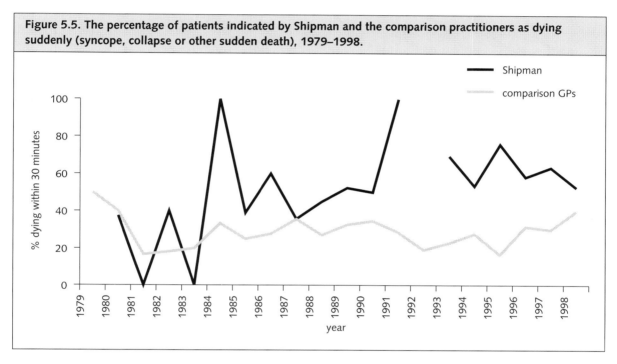

**Figure 5.5. The percentage of patients indicated by Shipman and the comparison practitioners as dying suddenly (syncope, collapse or other sudden death), 1979–1998.**

The terms syncope and collapse were used by both Shipman and the comparison practitioners to indicate that death was sudden. Shipman used one of these descriptions for the mode of death in 54.4% of cases, but the respective percentage for the comparison practitioners was only 24.2% (Table 5.11). The comparison practitioners were more likely to report that dying had taken longer, using the terms coma or exhaustion in 68.8% of cases. Figure 5.5 confirms that the proportion of deaths classified by the terms syncope or collapse as dying suddenly was relatively high throughout the period 1980–1998.

Form B requires the practitioner to indicate the basis for the observations made on the mode of death. Shipman was more likely to claim the observations as his own or his own supplemented by the observations of relatives, carers or other professionals (Table 5.12).

**Table 5.12. The source of observations on the mode of death recorded by Shipman and comparison practitioners.** ($X_6^2 = 20.5$; $p - 0.002$).

| Source of observations | Shipman | | Comparison GPs | |
|---|---|---|---|---|
| | N | % | N | % |
| own | 75 | 25.7 | 82 | 17.3 |
| own plus other professionals | 14 | 4.8 | 47 | 9.9 |
| own plus carers or relatives | 110 | 37.7 | 152 | 32.0 |
| other professionals | 11 | 3.8 | 28 | 5.9 |
| relatives or carers | 81 | 27.7 | 165 | 34.7 |
| other | 1 | 0.3 | 1 | 0.2 |
| total | 292 | | 475 | |

In response to this question, Shipman frequently gave additional details about the circumstances of the death. The following are a selection of such comments made on cremation forms between 1984 and 1998:

- *seen by self 11.30. neighbour saw patient at 13.00 found at 15.00 by self and neighbour*

- *seen 2 hours before death with ct, atrial fibrillation & PND; found in chair by neighbour*

- *own, seen at 15.00 found by relative about 16.00*

- *saw patient at home, diagnosis made, arranged admission ambulance, patient dead when went back, all within 10 mins.*

Comments were also recorded in response to the question about persons present at death, for example:

- *no one, seen at 15.30 found at 16.00*

- *no one other than self*

- *no one seen by me 13.00 found by relative 14.30.*

The cremation forms contained information about several of the features found in the cases for which Shipman was convicted of murder, for example, time and place of death, suddenness of death and whether Shipman was present or had seen the patient shortly before death. Therefore, it was possible to classify cases on the basis of information recorded on the cremation forms into highly suspicious, moderately suspicious or not suspicious. However, although clinical records contain sufficient information to enable a view to be formed about the relationship between certified cause of death and clinical history, cremation forms do not. Of the 292 deaths, 177 (60.6%) were classified as moderately or highly suspicious (Table 5.13).

**Table 5.13 The proportion of cases classified on the information on cremation forms into highly, moderately or not suspicious.** (males vs females: $X_2^2 = 13.4$; $p - 0.001$).

| Level of suspicion | number | Females (%) |
|---|---|---|
| none | 115 (39.4) | 68 (59.1) |
| moderate | 41 (14.0) | 27 (65.9) |
| high | 136 (46.6) | 109 (80.1) |

Among those classified as highly suspicious, the proportion that were female was higher than in the moderately or not suspicious groups, although the deaths of 27 males were classified as highly suspicious and 14 as moderately suspicious. There was no difference in mean age between patients classified in different levels of suspicion. Death was more likely to occur at home in those cases classified as suspicious (Table 5.14).

| Table 5.14. The place of deaths classified as highly, moderately or not suspicious. Deaths taking place elsewhere include those in residential or nursing homes and one death that occurred in the street. ($X^2_8 = 89.0$; $p - 0.000$). | | | | |
|---|---|---|---|---|
| Level of suspicion | Home | Practice | Elsewhere | Total |
| none | 61  (27.0) | | 54  (88.5) | 115 |
| moderate | 35  (15.5) | | 6  (9.8) | 42 |
| high | 130  (57.5) | 5  (100) | 1  (1.6) | 136 |
| | 226  (100) | 5  (100) | 61  (100) | 292 |

The proportion of deaths each year that were classified as moderately or highly suspicious varied from 0 to 100%, but cases throughout the period were identified as suspicious (Figure 5.6).

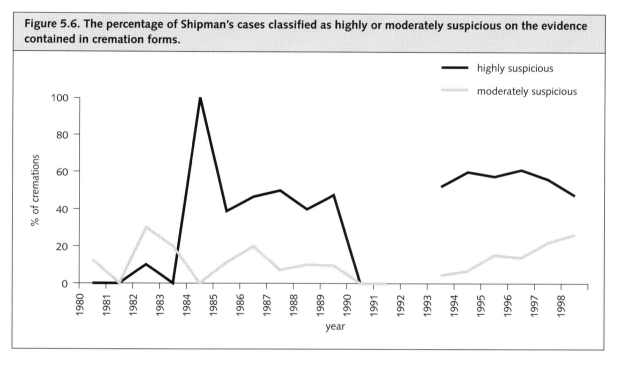

Figure 5.6. The percentage of Shipman's cases classified as highly or moderately suspicious on the evidence contained in cremation forms.

Of the 499 deaths for which Shipman issued MCCDs when working in Hyde, some documentary evidence was available from either records or cremation forms for 317 (63.5%). 168 (53.0%) of these were classified as highly suspicious, 47 (14.8%) as moderately suspicious, and 102 (32.2%) as not suspicious.

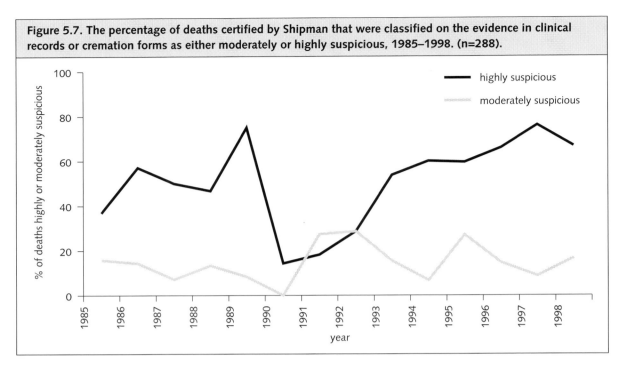

**Figure 5.7. The percentage of deaths certified by Shipman that were classified on the evidence in clinical records or cremation forms as either moderately or highly suspicious, 1985–1998. (n=288).**

Figure 5.7 shows the proportion of deaths certified by Shipman that were classified on review of records of cremation forms into highly or moderately suspicious for each year 1985–1998. The years before 1985 have been omitted since documentary evidence is available for only a few cases. The pattern reflects that shown in Figure 5.6, which contains data from cremation forms only. In most years, a high proportion were classified as either highly or moderately suspicious, although the proportion fell steeply in 1990 at the same time as the total annual number of deaths fell. The proportion rose again in 1993, at the same time as the total annual number of deaths increased.

## Form C

It is usual practice for the practitioner completing Form B to contact another practitioner, generally by telephone, to discuss the circumstances of the death. If the second practitioner is willing to complete Form C, he or she will make an external inspection of the body prior to completing the form. The doctors who gave evidence at the trial about the completion of Form C all reported following these routine procedures. They received details of the patient's clinical history and terminal illness from Shipman, and undertook an external examination of the body. In one of the convictions, Shipman reported showing his records to the doctor asked to complete Form C. In all cases reviewed in the audit, the general practitioner reported that they agreed with the certified cause of death.

Shipman was the practitioner completing Form C in 56 of the 767 cases included in the audit. Forty-eight other practitioners had also completed Form C. Of the 292 Form Bs completed by Shipman, 19 practitioners completed one or more Form Cs. The numbers completed by different general practitioners would have been influenced by the period during which the practitioner worked in Hyde, and the locality of their practices and the patients. No practitioner who had been a partner of Shipman prior to 1992 completed a Form C either before or after 1992. The practitioner completing the highest number of Form Cs for Shipman signed 44, followed in descending order by practitioners who signed 43, 33, 31, 29, 23, 18, 17, 14 and 11. Ten practitioners completed fewer than 10 forms each.

In coming to a view about the circumstances of the death, the practitioner may seek additional information from the deceased's relatives, carers or other professionals who had been in attendance.

In almost all cases, the practitioner did not seek any corroborative evidence from these sources. The only practitioner who sought additional evidence with any regularity was Shipman (Table 5.15).

| Table 5.15. Numbers of cases in which Shipman and other doctors completing Form C sought additional corroborative evidence about the circumstances of deaths from general practice or hospital notes, or other persons including relatives or other health professionals. ($X_3^2 = 23.8$; $p - 0.000$). | | | | |
|---|---|---|---|---|
| | Shipman | | Comparison GPs | |
| | N | % | N | % |
| no additional information sought | 18 | 32.1 | 705 | 99.2 |
| review of GP notes | 26 | 46.4 | 0 | 0 |
| review of hospital records | 9 | 16.1 | 0 | 0 |
| discussion with another person | 3 | 5.4 | 6 | 0.8 |
| Total | 56 | | 711 | |

# 5.4 Conclusions

There were distinct differences between Shipman and the comparison practitioners in the information they recorded on cremation Form B. These differences were typical of those associated with the convictions, in that among Shipman's patients, a higher proportion died at home, they were more likely to be female, to die in the afternoon, die suddenly, and allegedly from strokes, heart conditions or old age. Furthermore, these differences were discernable from 1985 onwards, the year from which all the cremations forms had been retained. It is notable that in those years with relatively high numbers of deaths, the proportions classified as highly or moderately suspicious were also relatively high.

It was notable that Shipman took particular care to obtain corroborative information when completing Form C. It is possible only to speculate on his motives, but his habit points to an action that could form a component of revised procedures for death certification – the review of corroborating evidence.

In the absence of an adequate system to record and monitor the numbers and circumstances of deaths, the detection of Shipman's high numbers of deaths was dependent on the chance of observations of individual practitioners or medical referees. It may be asked whether the medical referees of crematoria, or the practitioners completing Form C, should have been able to detect the relatively high number of deaths among Shipman's patients. In fact, the concerns of an undertaker and a local practitioner did lead to an initial police investigation. However, it should be remembered that medical referees deal with large numbers of cremations each year (see Table 5.1). In the absence of an efficient recording system, they only have their own memories to help them detect patterns and numbers of deaths.

A similar problem faces practitioners completing Form C. Since Shipman was able to ask several different practitioners to complete Form C, no single practitioner would automatically be exposed to an excess number of patient deaths. In these circumstances, if any practitioner did notice an excess, it could readily and credibly be ascribed to factors such as Shipman's large list or his alleged preference to care for patients in their own homes in their final illnesses.

# Six: Cases referred to the Coroner

## 6.1 Background

The main duty of a coroner is to enquire into certain deaths occurring in his jurisdiction (Devis and Rooney, 1999). The coroner is appointed by a local authority such as a county council, metropolitan borough or London borough. A registrar must refer a death to the coroner (unless it has already been reported) if it falls into one of the following categories:

- the deceased was not attended during the last illness by a doctor;

- the registrar has been unable to obtain a completed death certificate, or it appears the deceased was not seen by the certifying doctor either after death or during the 14 days before death;

- the cause of death appears to be unknown;

- the registrar has reason to believe the death was unnatural, or caused by violence, neglect, abortion or was in any way suspicious;

- the death occurred during an operation or before recovery from an anaesthetic;

- the death was due to industrial disease or industrial poisoning.

Doctors may voluntarily refer deaths to the coroner, and should consider whether the death was an accident, a suicide, whether it occurred during or shortly after detention in police or prison custody, whether there is uncertainty about the cause of death, and whether the doctor is legally qualified to certify death. Deaths for which no doctor is in attendance, such as unexpected or violent deaths may be referred directly to the coroner by the police.

The coroner has three principal options in response to a referral. If satisfied that the death is due to natural causes, the coroner will instruct the registrar to register the death.

Enquiries may also be received from doctors, for example when the doctor has not seen the deceased person within 14 days before death. If satisfied about the cause of death, the coroner will authorise the doctor to issue a certificate. The first officer and secretary from the coroner's office in Stockport gave evidence at the trial. They confirmed that they took calls from local doctors wanting to report a death or discuss a particular case. They made clear that if a general practitioner contacted the office merely to seek advice before a certificate was issued, they would not necessarily make a record of the call. They also confirmed that the criteria for determining whether a certificate could be issued were the doctor having seen the patient within fourteen days and the medical history reflecting the cause of death. For example, if the doctor had attended the patient within the fourteen day period and said that the patient had died of old age, having deteriorated over a period of time, the doctor would be advised that a certificate could be issued and the coroner's office would not need to be involved.

The second option available to the coroner is to request a post-mortem examination, most commonly when the cause of death is unknown. It should be noted that during the trial, evidence was presented that in many of the cases considered, Shipman had advised relatives that post mortems were not required and that he could issue a MCCD. If the post mortem shows that the cause of death was natural, the coroner may issue a certificate of cause of death (Form 100B). The registrar will use this certificate to register the death. An inquest is the third option open to the coroner. If an inquest is held, a certificate (Form 99(REV)) is issued after the inquest by the coroner.

A potential explanation for the excess number of deaths certified by Shipman is that he did not make referrals to the coroner. If patients die suddenly, due to natural causes, it could be argued that he would issue a MCCD in order to relieve the relative of any distress that a post mortem examination might cause. Conversely, it was argued at the trial by the prosecution that Shipman told relatives that post mortem examinations were not required to reduce the risk that his murderous activities would be detected. It is also possible that some patients who had not died of natural causes had been confirmed dead by doctors other than Shipman, for example locums, general practitioners on duty out of hours, or hospital doctors. In these cases, referral to the coroner could have resulted in a post mortem at which no clear cause of death would be found. In the light of what is now known, such cases should be regarded as suspicious. Therefore, an audit of the referrals to the coroner was undertaken to determine the extent to which Shipman made referrals to the coroner.

## 6.2 Methods

Stockport coroner, Mr John Pollard, agreed to the review of records of cases referred to the coroner's office during Shipman's working life in Hyde. Records were available for all years from 1977. Table 6.1 shows the annual numbers of cases handled by the coroner throughout this period. Each year, approximately 2,500 deaths were investigated.

| year | post-mortem | Inquests not held | | Inquests held | | Total deaths investigated | |
|------|-------------|------|--------|------|--------|------|--------|
| | | male | female | male | female | male | female |
| 1977 | Yes | 890 | 745 | 131 | 89 | 1021 | 834 |
| | No | 299 | 268 | – | – | 299 | 268 |
| | Total | 1189 | 1013 | 131 | 89 | 1320 | 1102 |
| 1978 | Yes | 878 | 743 | 144 | 106 | 1022 | 849 |
| | No | 333 | 283 | – | – | 333 | 283 |
| | Total | 1211 | 1026 | 144 | 106 | 1355 | 1132 |
| 1979 | Yes | 971 | 840 | 134 | 111 | 1105 | 951 |
| | No | 334 | 291 | – | – | 334 | 291 |
| | Total | 1305 | 1131 | 134 | 111 | 1439 | 1242 |
| 1980 | Yes | 940 | 822 | 126 | 120 | 1066 | 942 |
| | No | 294 | 326 | – | – | 294 | 326 |
| | Total | 1234 | 1148 | 126 | 120 | 1360 | 1268 |
| 1981 | Yes | 917 | 799 | 135 | 99 | 1052 | 898 |
| | No | 365 | 357 | – | – | 365 | 357 |
| | Total | 1282 | 1156 | 135 | 99 | 1417 | 1255 |
| 1982 | Yes | 1041 | 780 | 107 | 90 | 1148 | 870 |
| | No | 311 | 340 | – | – | 311 | 340 |
| | Total | 1352 | 1120 | 107 | 90 | 1459 | 1210 |
| 1983 | Yes | 985 | 855 | 142 | 104 | 1127 | 870 |
| | No | 369 | 352 | – | – | 311 | 340 |
| | Total | 1354 | 1207 | 142 | 104 | 1459 | 1210 |
| 1984 | Yes | 940 | 779 | 121 | 79 | 1061 | 858 |
| | No | 340 | 341 | – | – | 340 | 341 |
| | Total | 1280 | 1120 | 121 | 79 | 1401 | 1199 |

Table 6.1. The annual numbers of cases investigated by the Stockport coroner, 1977–99.

| Table 6.1. continued | | | | | | | |
|---|---|---|---|---|---|---|---|
| | | Inquests not held | | Inquests held | | Total deaths investigated | |
| year | post-mortem | male | female | male | female | male | female |
| 1985 | Yes | 954 | 786 | 127 | 58 | 1081 | 844 |
| | No | 332 | 343 | – | – | 332 | 343 |
| | Total | 1286 | 1129 | 127 | 58 | 1413 | 1187 |
| 1986 | Yes | 934 | 761 | 137 | 100 | 1071 | 861 |
| | No | 354 | 381 | – | – | 354 | 381 |
| | Total | 1288 | 1142 | 137 | 100 | 1425 | 1242 |
| 1987 | Yes | 808 | 681 | 145 | 67 | 953 | 748 |
| | No | 364 | 406 | – | – | 364 | 406 |
| | Total | 1172 | 1087 | 145 | 67 | 1317 | 1154 |
| 1988 | Yes | 800 | 640 | 143 | 81 | 943 | 721 |
| | No | 390 | 449 | – | – | 390 | 449 |
| | Total | 1190 | 1089 | 143 | 81 | 1333 | 1170 |
| 1989* | Yes | | | | | | |
| | No | | | | | | |
| | Total | | | | | | |
| 1990** | Yes | 337 | 282 | 54 | 21 | 391 | 303 |
| | No | 140 | 166 | – | – | 140 | 166 |
| | Total | 448 | 448 | 54 | 21 | 531 | 469 |
| 1991 | Yes | 766 | 634 | 136 | 74 | 902 | 708 |
| | No | 333 | 359 | – | – | 333 | 359 |
| | Total | 1099 | 993 | 136 | 74 | 1235 | 1067 |
| 1992 | Yes | 794 | 672 | 112 | 63 | 906 | 735 |
| | No | 286 | 369 | – | – | 286 | 369 |
| | Total | 1080 | 1041 | 112 | 63 | 1192 | 1104 |
| 1993 | Yes | 794 | 694 | 140 | 57 | 934 | 751 |
| | No | 364 | 458 | – | – | 364 | 458 |
| | Total | 1158 | 1152 | 140 | 57 | 1298 | 1209 |
| 1994 | Yes | 797 | 680 | 154 | 63 | 951 | 743 |
| | No | 406 | 436 | – | – | 406 | 436 |
| | Total | 1203 | 1116 | 154 | 63 | 1357 | 1179 |
| 1995 | Yes | 838 | 711 | 162 | 71 | 1000 | 782 |
| | No | 388 | 469 | – | – | 388 | 469 |
| | Total | 1226 | 1180 | 162 | 71 | 1388 | 1251 |
| 1996 | Yes | 825 | 752 | 190 | 86 | 1015 | 838 |
| | No | 434 | 449 | – | – | 434 | 449 |
| | Total | 1259 | 1201 | 190 | 86 | 1449 | 1287 |
| 1997 | Yes | 823 | 710 | 187 | 121 | 1010 | 831 |
| | No | 381 | 502 | – | – | 381 | 502 |
| | Total | 1204 | 1212 | 187 | 121 | 1391 | 1333 |
| 1998 | Yes | 954 | 913 | 222 | 105 | 1176 | 1018 |
| | No | 326 | 374 | – | – | 326 | 374 |
| | Total | 1280 | 1287 | 222 | 105 | 1502 | 1392 |
| 1999 | Yes | 858 | 887 | 226 | 137 | 1084 | 1024 |
| | No | 277 | 345 | 1 | – | 278 | 345 |
| | Total | 1135 | 1232 | 227 | 137 | 1362 | 1369 |

* data for 1989 not available
** data for 1990 only available for six months.

The record system consisted of carefully indexed and stored paper records, each case being assigned a unique code number. From 1997, a computer system was also used. A search of the computer file had been undertaken during the police investigation (January 1997 to September 1998), and one case referred by Shipman had been identified.

From the 22 years concerned (1977–1998), a sample of five was reviewed – 1978, 1982, 1987, 1992, 1996. 1997 and 1998 were excluded since the computer search had been undertaken. 1977 was excluded since this was Shipman's first year in Hyde and he worked for only part of the year. The sample was taken to ensure a spread between 1978 and 1996. All paper files for these years (total 12,659) were hand searched to identify deaths of patients recorded as being registered patients of Shipman or the comparison group of general practitioners. Thus, patients who died in hospital or were referred to the coroner by another doctor or by a police officer were included. In addition, patients who were recorded as having been seen after death by these doctors were also included.

In the case of sudden death at home, the general practitioner asked to attend may be the deceased's own general practitioner, a partner of the practitioner, or a locum or deputising doctor. If the attending doctor can determine that the patient has not been under the care of a doctor, a direct referral to the coroner is generally arranged. In some cases it may not be clear whether the patient was under the care of a doctor, and the attending doctor will contact the patient's regular general practitioner to determine whether that practitioner is able to issue a certificate, or whether a referral to the coroner is required. In a proportion of cases, patients who collapse will be admitted to hospital, but die shortly afterwards. In these circumstances, the hospital doctor often contacts the patient's general practitioner to determine whether the practitioner is able to issue a certificate. If not, a referral to the coroner is made.

Thus, those patients of Shipman who died suddenly may have been be referred to the coroner by Shipman himself if he had not been attending the patient recently or did not know the cause of death, by a hospital doctor if the patient died in hospital, or a police officer, or by another doctor attending the deceased in the community. In those cases referred by someone other than Shipman, a discussion may have taken place between Shipman and the referring person, but no documentary record of these discussions is available. Indeed, it is generally not possible to be certain of the source of referrals from the paper records. If a referral is made, a form is completed by a coroner's officer to record preliminary details including the name of the patient's general practitioner, and the name of any doctor seeing the patient after death. In the audit, it has been assumed that in most cases the referral was initiated by the doctor who saw the patient after death. However, this may not always have been the case, since any discussions between the attending practitioner and the general practitioner are not recorded.

Information was collected about the patients of Shipman and the comparison general practitioners. The details about each case collected from the coroner's records included the patient's general practitioner, whether an inquest had been held or a post mortem undertaken, and the determined cause of death.

# 6.3 Findings

The numbers of patients of Shipman and the comparison practitioners whose deaths were investigated by Stockport coroner are shown in Table 6.2. Table 6.3 presents information about the person most likely to have initiated the referral of the patients included in Table 6.2.

**Table 6.2. The numbers of patients of Shipman and the comparison general practitioners whose deaths were investigated by the coroner by means of inquests, post mortems or investigations without post mortem.**

| Year | Category | General practitioners | | | | | | |
|------|----------|---------|---|---|---|---|---|---|
|      |          | Shipman | 1 | 2 | 3 | 4 | 5 | 6 |
| 1978 | inquest  | 4  | 1  |    |    |   |   |   |
|      | PM       | 6  | 7  | 8  | 5  | 1 |   |   |
|      | no PM    |    |    | 1  |    |   |   |   |
|      | total    | 10 | 8  | 9  | 5  | 1 |   |   |
| 1982 | inquest  | 2  |    | 2  |    |   |   |   |
|      | PM       | 7  | 4  | 9  | 9  | 1 |   |   |
|      | no PM    | 1  | 2  | 1  | 1  |   | 1 |   |
|      | total    | 10 | 6  | 12 | 10 | 1 | 1 |   |
| 1987 | inquest  | 1  | 1  |    | 1  |   | 1 |   |
|      | PM       | 9  | 3  | 10 | 7  | 6 | 4 |   |
|      | no PM    |    |    |    |    |   |   |   |
|      | total    | 10 | 4  | 10 | 8  | 6 | 5 |   |
| 1992 | inquest  | 1  | 2  |    |    | 1 | 1 | 1 |
|      | PM       | 2  | 8  | 7  | 5  | 7 | 3 |   |
|      | no PM    |    |    |    |    |   |   |   |
|      | total    | 3  | 10 | 7  | 5  | 8 | 4 | 1 |
| 1996 | inquest  | 1  | 1  | 1  |    |   |   |   |
|      | PM       | 2  | 3  | 3  |    | 5 | 4 | 4 |
|      | no PM    |    |    |    |    |   |   |   |
|      | total    | 3  | 4  | 4  | 0  | 5 | 4 | 4 |

Some were referred by hospital doctors in the case of deaths of people shortly after admission to hospital, and many of these were found at post mortem to have been due to ischaemic heart disease. A smaller proportion of deaths in hospital followed surgical operations. Other deaths were referred by police officers. These cases involved violent death due to accidents, house fires, or homicide.

Sudden deaths at home were usually referred by general practitioners or their deputising services, and most of these were investigated by post mortem examinations. Ischaemic heart disease was the most common finding. It is clear from Table 6.3 that in most years, Shipman did initiate referrals to the coroner and that his rate of referral was similar to the comparison practitioners (in Table 6.3, "GP" indicates that the patient was attended after death by their usual general practitioner, and that this practitioner had probably initiated the referral to the coroner).

**Table 6.3. Patients of Shipman and the comparison practitioners, indicating the probable person initiating the referral to the coroner. GP = own GP, other GP = partner of the general practitioner, locum, deputising doctor.**

| Year | Attended after death by | General practitioners | | | | | | |
|------|-------------------------|---------|---|---|---|---|---|---|
|      |                         | Shipman | 1 | 2 | 3 | 4 | 5 | 6 |
| 1978 | GP       | 3  |    | 1  |    |   |   |   |
|      | other GP | 3  | 3  | 4  | 1  |   |   |   |
|      | hospital | 1  | 4  | 1  | 4  |   |   |   |
|      | unknown  | 3  | 1  | 3  |    | 1 |   |   |
|      | total    | 10 | 8  | 9  | 5  | 1 |   |   |
| 1982 | GP       | 4  |    | 4  | 5  |   | 1 |   |
|      | other GP | 5  | 3  | 5  | 4  | 1 |   |   |
|      | hospital | 1  | 1  | 1  |    |   |   |   |
|      | unknown  |    | 2  | 12 | 1  |   |   |   |
|      | total    | 10 | 6  | 12 | 10 | 1 | 1 |   |
| 1987 | GP       | 3  |    | 2  | 3  | 1 | 1 |   |
|      | other GP | 3  | 1  | 4  | 1  | 1 | 1 |   |
|      | hospital | 4  | 2  | 4  | 3  | 4 | 3 |   |
|      | unknown  |    | 1  |    | 1  |   |   |   |
|      | total    | 10 | 4  | 10 | 8  | 6 | 5 |   |
| 1992 | GP       |    | 2  | 4  | 1  | 1 |   |   |
|      | other GP |    | 2  | 1  |    | 3 | 2 |   |
|      | hospital | 2  | 4  | 2  | 4  | 3 | 1 |   |
|      | unknown  | 1  | 2  |    |    | 1 | 1 | 1 |
|      | total    | 3  | 10 | 7  | 5  | 8 | 4 | 1 |
| 1996 | GP       | 2  | 1  |    |    | 1 | 1 |   |
|      | other GP |    | 1  | 1  |    |   |   |   |
|      | hospital | 1  | 2  | 2  |    | 4 | 2 | 3 |
|      | unknown  |    |    | 1  |    |   | 1 | 1 |
|      | total    | 3  | 4  | 4  | 0  | 5 | 4 | 4 |

## Inquests

In the years included in the audit, the deaths of seven patients of Shipman were investigated by the coroner. Of the three in 1978, two were determined to be barbiturate overdoses and one died from bronchopneumonia following injuries caused by a road traffic accident. In 1982, the death of one patient of Shipman was investigated by inquest. This patient died from injuries sustained during a fall at home. In 1987, the death of one patient of Shipman was investigated. This case was referred to the coroner by Shipman because of the possibility of asbestosis. In 1992, one death of a patient of Shipman was investigated by an inquest, death occurring following a road traffic accident. One case was also the subject of an inquest in 1996. Shipman referred the death, indicating that he suspected that the patient may have committed suicide. The post mortem indicated the cause of death as being left ventricular failure and ischaemic heart disease, but because of Shipman's concern, a full set of toxicological tests was undertaken. The results were positive for propranolol only.

## Post mortems

During the five years included in the audit, the deaths of 26 of Shipman's patients were investigated by coroner's post mortems. The identified causes of death are summarised in Table 6.4. In each case, a specific diagnosis was confirmed.

| Table 6.4. Patients of Shipman referred to the coroner showing results of post mortem examinations. | |
|---|---|
| | **Cause of death determined by post mortem** |
| 1 | Bronchopneumonia; carcinoma of bronchus |
| 2 | Myocardial infarct; coronary atheroma |
| 3 | Left ventricular failure; ischaemic heart disease; mild hydronephrosis |
| 4 | Left ventricular failure; ischaemic heart disease |
| 5 | Left ventricular failure; ischaemic heart disease |
| 6 | Acute left ventricular failure; ischaemic heart disease; hypertensive heart disease |
| 7 | Subarachnoid haemorrhage |
| 8 | Coronary occlusion; coronary atherosclerosis |
| 9 | Sudden death in infancy syndrome |
| 10 | Cor pulmonale; bronchopneumonia; acute on chronic bronchitis with emphysema |
| 11 | Lobar pneumonia |
| 12 | Haemopericardium; rupture of the heart; myocardial infarction; coronary thrombosis |
| 13 | Status asthmaticus |
| 14 | Cardiac tamponade; intra pericardial haemorrhage; myocardial infarction with rupture of left ventricle |
| 15 | Haemopericardium; rupture of the heart due to myocardial infarction; coronary atheroma |
| 16 | Left ventricular failure; myocardial fibrosis with aneurysm of left ventricle; ischaemic heart disease |
| 17 | Left ventricular failure; ischaemic heart disease |
| 18 | Bronchopneumonia |
| 19 | Fatty metamorphosis of the liver |
| 20 | Myocardial infarction; coronary atheroma |
| 21 | Recent myocardial infarction; ischaemic heart disease |
| 22 | Subarachnoid haemorrhage; hypertensive heart disease |
| 23 | Carcinoma right lung with bronchopneumonia |
| 24 | Cor pulmonale; chronic bronchitis; emphysema with patchy bronchopneumonia |
| 25 | Coronary insufficiency; coronary atherosclerosis; bronchopneumonia |
| 26 | Left ventricular failure; ischaemic heart disease; suppurative bronchitis and bronchopneumonia |

# 6.4 Conclusions

This aspect of the audit was undertaken to determine whether Shipman avoided making referrals to the coroner or whether sudden deaths among his patients had been investigated by post mortem. The findings are essentially negative. They make clear that the excess number of deaths certified by Shipman cannot be explained as being due to failure to make referrals to the coroner. In most years investigated, Shipman had referred cases of sudden death to the coroner. Other doctors had also referred several of his patients who died suddenly. The post mortems undertaken all led to firm conclusions about the causes of death.

The deaths of seven of Shipman's patients were also investigated by inquests. Most were caused by accidents or overdoses, but one was referred by Shipman and detailed toxicological tests were undertaken because he claimed to suspect that the patient had committed suicide. The notes of this patient were available for review and did not contain a history indicating major depression or suicidal ideation, although the patient had recently suffered a bereavement.

It was possible to be confident about the source of referrals in most cases, but it should be noted that details about the source of referral were not always clear. This information is recorded by the coroner's officer and in the audit was generally assumed to be the doctor who confirmed the fact of death, unless a clear statement to the contrary had been made. In any review of the recording system, it would be appropriate to revise the form to record the source of referrals to the coroner.

# Seven: Restricted drugs

## 7.1 Background

The prescribing of certain drugs is restricted under the terms of the Misuse of Drugs Act 1971, the Misuse of Drugs Regulations, 1985, and the Misuse of Drugs (Supply to Addicts) Regulations, 1997. The classes of drugs subject to these regulations are shown in Box 6.1. The Regulations require that prescriptions for controlled drugs are written in the prescriber's own handwriting and state the name and address of the patient, the preparation and strength of the drug, the dose, and the total quantity to be dispensed in both words and figures. Drugs classified under schedule 2 of the Misuse of Drugs Regulations 1985 include diamorphine, morphine and pethidine. Doctors who hold a supply of these drugs must store them in a secure place, and must record in a register details about the purchase and administration of the drugs.

The misuse of Drugs Act 1971 includes specifications for registers. They should be bound and preserved for a minimum of two years, and should record the day on which drugs are obtained or supplied. Doctors must produce their registers on request by persons authorised by the Secretary of State. Such inspections used to be undertaken by the Medical Officers of the Regional Medical Service, but arrangements for routine inspection are now unclear. The Act also regulates arrangements for the destruction of any unused drugs, and subsequent regulations require that controlled drugs be stored in a locked receptacle.

Shipman was convicted of the murders of 15 patients, nine of whom had been buried. During the investigation by Greater Manchester Police, the bodies of these patients were exhumed and post mortem examinations undertaken. In each case, autopsy did not reveal a natural cause of death, and in particular did not confirm the causes of deaths as certified by Shipman. Toxicological tests were undertaken on samples of hair and thigh muscle of all nine patients, and on samples of liver in a small number of cases. The hair samples confirmed that all the patients could be regarded as 'morphine naïve', in other words they were not regular users of morphine. The thigh muscle and liver samples all revealed the presence of morphine in levels compatible with the administration of fatal doses, and in each case, the cause of death given by the Home Office Pathologist was morphine toxicity.

> **Box 6.1. Classes of drugs subject to restrictions.**
>
> The Misuse of Drugs Act 1971 defines three classes of drugs:
>
> A – alfentanil, cocaine, dextromoramide, diamorphine (heroin), dipipanone, lysergide (LSD), methadone, morphine, opium, pethidine, phencyclidine, and Class B substances when prepared for injection.
>
> B – oral amphetamines, barbiturates, cannabis, cannabis resin, codeine, ethylmorphine, glutethimide, pentazocine, phenmetrazine and pholcodine.
>
> C – certain drugs related to amphetamines such as benzphetamine and chlorphentermine, buprenorphine, diethylproprion, mazindol, meprobamate, pemoline, pipradrol, most benzodiazepines, androgenic and anabolic steroids, clenbuterol, chorionic gonadotrphin (HCG), non-human chorionic gonadotrophin, somatotrophin, somatrem and somatropin.
>
> The Misuse of Drugs Regulations 1985 defines those who are authorised to supply controlled drugs.
>
> Schedule 1 – cannabis, LSD etc which are not used medicinally. Possession and supply are prohibited except in accordance with Home Office authority.
>
> Schedule 2 – diamorphine, morphine, pethidine, secobarbital, glutethmide, amphetamine, cocaine; these are subject to the full controlled drug requirements relating to prescriptions, safe custody, need to keep registers etc.
>
> Schedule 3 – barbiturates, buprenorphine, diethylproprion, flunitrazepm, mazindol, meprobamate, pentazocine, phentermine and temazepam. These are subject to the special prescription requirements but not custody requirements nor the need to keep registers (subject to some exceptions).
>
> Schedule 4 – benzodiazepines, pemoline, androgenic and anabolic steroids, clenbuterol, chorionic gonadotrophin (HCG), non human chorionic gonadotrophin, somatotropin, somatrem, somatropin. Controlled drug prescription requirements do not apply, nor do safe custody requirements.
>
> Schedule 5 – those preparations that, because of their strength, are exempt from virtually all controlled drugs regulations.

During the trial, evidence was presented to show that Shipman had access to diamorphine that he could have used to murder patients. In a search of his house following his arrest, four 10mg ampoules of diamorphine were found, stored inside a box that had contained methotrimeprazine (Nozinan). Through reference to the batch number, it was established that the diamorphine medication had been prescribed to a patient of Shipman who had died over three years before. The records of this patient showed that ten 10mg ampoules remained unused after his death. Shipman claimed that he had destroyed the other six ampoules but could not explain why he had retained four.

Shipman did not maintain a controlled drugs register. He explained that he was aware of the regulations, but since 1976 had made it his policy not to keep controlled drugs and therefore did not need a register. He claimed that on the few occasions that controlled drugs were urgently required, he would write out a prescription in the patient's name and collect it immediately from a pharmacy. Thus, no controlled drugs register is available for investigation of Shipman's prescribing of these drugs.

Greater Manchester Police inspected the controlled drugs registers maintained by five pharmacies in Hyde. They found that at no time had Shipman signed orders or requisitions for controlled drugs. Several patients gave evidence at the trial relating to the prescribing and administration of morphine and diamorphine. Shipman had administered morphine to one patient without issuing a prescription in the name of the patient, indicating that he did have morphine in his possession. In one case, Shipman admitted carrying diamorphine that he had administered to a patient. In another case, he had written a prescription for diamorphine and presented it to a pharmacy himself, but there was no record that the drug had been administered to the patient. On other occasions, Shipman had signed prescriptions for controlled drugs dated after the death of the patients concerned.

Pharmacy staff gave evidence that to their knowledge Shipman had never returned unused drugs for destruction. However, it was established that he had collected unused controlled drugs following the deaths of patients at home. He claimed that he destroyed these drugs but this assertion was challenged by the evidence of other witnesses. The discovery in Shipman's home of ampoules of diamorphine left unused after the death of a patient has been referred to above. Evidence was also presented that many of Shipman's prescriptions for diamorphine were for doses of 30mg, even though the patients had not received diamorphine previously, and would be unable to tolerate such a high dose. Shipman explained that he only administered part of the dose and discarded the remainder, agreeing that he had got into a bad habit of prescribing 30mg. Shipman also agreed that it was an offence under the Misuse of Drugs Act to fail to make a record of the administration of a controlled drug to a patient, and also accepted that in one case he had failed to make such a record.

# 7.2 Methods

Since no comprehensive record of Shipman's prescribing throughout his working life was available, three principal sources were used. The Prescription Pricing Authority (PPA) provides routine data about the prescribing patterns of general practitioners to Health Authorities, and these data were used to review Shipman's general prescribing patterns from January 1995 to October 1998. Second, the PPA had identified all prescriptions issued by Shipman between May 1997 and October 1998. Third, pharmacies are required to maintain registers of the dispensing of controlled drugs, and therefore these registers were reviewed.

### General Prescribing Patterns

The PPA retains prescribing data in electronic form for a period of up to three years, after which it is archived to tape. However, the data that had been sent to West Pennine Health Authority relating to the period 1995–1998 were readily available. Prescribing reports sent by PPA to Health Authorities are in a standard form, referred to as Prescribing Analysis and Costs (PACT). The quarterly version is issued automatically to all general practitioners for the quarters ending March, June, September and December. Full details are sent to Authorities in electronic form – electronic PACT (PPA, 1994). The data are used by Health Authorities and Primary Care Groups to identify practitioners or practices with atypical prescribing patterns so that they can be offered help and encouragement to improve if necessary. PACT can provide information about the numbers and costs of prescriptions, the drugs being grouped into classes in accordance with the system used in the British National Formulary. However, the data do not include information that identifies the patient, and therefore it is not possible to monitor the prescriptions issued to a particular patient over a period of time.

For the purposes of the audit, the PACT data held by West Pennine Health Authority were reviewed. Shipman's prescribing was compared to that of other practitioners in Tameside, with a particular focus on his prescribing of analgesics and drugs for cardiovascular disorders.

### Prescribing May 1997 – October 1998

The PPA undertook a search of all Shipman's prescriptions issued between May 1997 and October 1998. Although he was arrested on 7th September 1998, some of his prescriptions would have been dispensed after his arrest. However, the prescriptions issued after 7th September will also include those issued by locums. The PPA identified all those prescriptions for diamorphine, morphine and pethidine, including both oral and injection forms of these medications. They also identified prescriptions for methotrimeprazine that is used as an adjunct during terminal illness, and midazolam (Hypnovel).

### Controlled Drugs Registers in Pharmacies

Several pharmacies that served the population of Hyde were visited in order to inspect their controlled drugs registers. The pharmacies were those identified from the PPA data as having dispensed controlled drugs prescribed by Shipman from May 1997 – October 1998.

Six pharmacies identified in this way were visited. An additional pharmacy was also visited since it was the only principal local pharmacy that had not been identified in the PPA data file. The visits were undertaken in collaboration with the local inspector of the Royal Pharmaceutical Society.

# 7.3 Findings

### General Prescribing Patterns

A detailed report of the findings is included in Appendix Three, and only the key findings are discussed here. Shipman was the most costly prescriber in Tameside in terms of the cost of individual drugs, but the number of prescriptions he issued was close to the average for Tameside. His costs were particularly high for antihypertensive and lipid lowering drugs, but he did not prescribe antiplatlet drugs such as aspirin or dipyridamole as frequently as other local practitioners. His prescribing of analgesic drugs (BNF Section 4.7) was not substantially different to the prescribing of local colleagues.

### Prescribing May 1997 – October 1998

The numbers of prescriptions issued by Shipman for oral or injectable preparations of morphine, diamorphine, methotrimeprazine and midazolam are shown in Tables 7.1 and 7.2.

| Table 7.1. Numbers of prescriptions for oral or transdermal preparations of morphine, pethidine and methotrimeprazine, issued by Shipman between May 1997 and September 1998. | |
| --- | --- |
| **Medication** | **Number of prescriptions** |
| Oramorph oral solution 10mg/5ml | 10 |
| Oramorph oral solution 10mg/5ml Ud | 4 |
| MST Continus tabs 10mg | 47 |
| MST Continus tabs 15mg | 1 |
| MST Continus tabs 30 mg | 39 |
| MST Continus tabs 60 mg | 5 |
| MST Continus tabs 100mg | 3 |
| Durogesic patches 75mg | 1 |
| Durogesic patches 100mg | 1 |
| MXL cap 60mg | 1 |
| MXL cap 90mg | 1 |
| MXL cap 120mg | 7 |
| Pethidine tabs 50mg | 10 |
| Sevredol tab 50mg | 1 |
| Methotrimeprazine tab 25mg | 2 |

| Table 7.2. Numbers of prescriptions for morphine, diamorphine, methotrimeprazine and midazolam injections issued by Shipman, May 1997 – September 1998. | |
| --- | --- |
| **Medication** | **Number of prescriptions** |
| diamorphine 100mg with methotrimeprazine 2.5% 1ml | 6 |
| diamorphine 100mg | 4 |
| diamorphine 10mg | 7 |
| diamorphine 100mg with midazolam 5mg/ml | 1 |
| diamorphine 100mg with Stesolid soln 4mg/ml 2.5 ml rectal | 1 |
| diamorphine 30mg with methotrimeprazine 2.5 % 1ml | 1 |

On the basis of clinical judgement, the findings do not suggest that Shipman was issuing large numbers of prescriptions for diamorphine during this period. His use of methotrimeprazine was unremarkable and only one prescription for diamorphine was accompanied by a prescription for midazolam.

## Controlled Drugs Registers in Pharmacies

All the pharmacies had appropriately maintained controlled drugs registers, and used the versions originally published by the National Pharmaceutical Association. Some pharmacies had stored their registers beyond the legally required period, and registers at two pharmacies were available from 1977, another from 1981, a fourth from 1985, two others from 1994, and the seventh from 1992. Shipman's practice was sited next door to the pharmacy that had information available from 1992. This was the pharmacy used by most of Shipman's patients, and the register had been retained by Greater Manchester Police, who gave permission for its review in the audit.

The prescriptions for diamorphine injections are shown in Table 7.3. Most were dispensed by the pharmacy next door to the practice (pharmacy 1). The only unusual finding is that in 1993, 12 patients were issued prescriptions for single doses of 30mg of diamorphine injections. One patient was recorded as being issued two prescriptions, each for a single dose, and another patient received a prescription for ten ampoules of diamorphine 30 mg injection.

| Table 7.3. Prescriptions issued by Shipman for diamorphine injection. | | | | | |
|---|---|---|---|---|---|
| Year | Pharmacy | Medication | Number of patients | Number of prescriptions | Total number of ampoules |
| 1992 | 1 | Diamorphine 30mg | 1 | 1 | 1 |
| 1993 | 1 | Diamorphine 30mg | 14 | 15 | 26 |
| | | Diamorphine 100mg | 1 | 2 | 35 |
| 1994 | 1 | Diamorphine 100mg | 2 | 2 | 15 |
| | 6 | Diamorphine 10mg | 1 | 1 | 10 |
| 1995 | 1 | Diamorphine 10 mg | 2 | 5 | 50 |
| | | Diamorphine 30mg | 1 | 2 | 20 |
| | | Diamorphine 100mg | 5 | 8 | 53 |
| 1996 | 1 | Diamorphine 100mg | 2 | 23 | 343 |
| | | Diamorphine 500mg | 1 | 8 | 95 |
| 1997 | 1 | Diamorphine 10mg | 1 | 4 | 130 |
| | | Diamorphine 100mg | 4 | 9 | 100 |
| 1998 | 1 | Diamorphine 10mg | 1 | 1 | 10 |
| | | Diamorphine 100mg | 3 | 3 | 25 |
| | 4 | Diamorphine 10mg | 1 | 4 | 20 |
| | | Diamorphine 100mg | 1 | 1 | 10 |

No entries for morphine or Cyclimorph injections were found in any of the controlled drugs registers of the seven pharmacies, although Shipman had reported in his clinical records that he had administered these drugs to some patients. Only three of the pharmacies had records of dispensing prescriptions issued by Shipman for diamorphine injections. The pharmacies had dispensed prescriptions for a variety of oral opiate medication, including dipipanone (Diconal) morphine sulphate solution, MST Continus tablets, MXL capsules, pethidine, and dextromoramide (Palfium). There was no record of Shipman issuing a prescription for methadone, or for issuing prescriptions to people addicted to methadone or other opiates.

# 7.4 Conclusions

It was established during the trial that Shipman had access to diamorphine by taking possession of unused drugs following the deaths of patients nursed at home, or by writing prescriptions for diamorphine that he did not subsequently administer to the patient. The findings of the audit do not add substantially to this information.

Shipman's habit of prescribing single doses of diamorphine which he did not administer appears to have been restricted to 1993. In subsequent years, relatively small numbers of patients were recorded as receiving prescriptions for diamorphine, although several received large quantities during terminal care. No information about Shipman's prescribing of diamorphine injections prior to 1992 could be obtained.

None of the pharmacies that had stored their controlled drugs register relating to the earlier years had dispensed any diamorphine injections prescribed by Shipman.

The failure to find in the controlled drugs registers a record of morphine or Cyclimorph injections dispensed by a pharmacist on a prescription issued by Shipman raises the possibility that he may have obtained these drugs from other pharmacies or other sources. However, in the record of prescriptions prepared by the PPA for the period May 1997 to October 1998, no other pharmacy handled any of Shipman's prescriptions for diamorphine. All the pharmacies that had issued diamorphine were visited. Therefore, it cannot be ruled out that prior to 1997, other pharmacies not identified by the PPA data had dispensed prescriptions for diamorphine or other opiates issued by Shipman.

In the years following 1993, Shipman appears to have obtained diamorphine by taking possession of unused medication following the deaths of patients at home. This conclusion is consistent with the discovery by Greater Manchester Police of diamorphine in Shipman's home that was identified as having been dispensed for a patient who died three years before.

Although it is clear that Shipman had access to diamorphine and had diamorphine in his possession, it is difficult to determine how much diamorphine he may have unlawfully possessed. Therefore, it is impossible to show that Shipman obtained all the diamorphine required to administer lethal doses to all the cases classified as suspicious. Furthermore, there is no record of his prescribing of diamorphine prior to 1992.

The audit indicates several deficiencies in current systems to monitor the prescribing of controlled drugs. Shipman was able to practise as a general practitioner without using – or being required to explain his failure to use – a controlled drugs register. Arrangements to monitor general practitioners' controlled drugs registers require review. Inspectors of the Royal Pharmaceutical Society are empowered under the Misuse of Drugs Act 1971 to inspect the controlled drugs registers maintained in pharmacies. Clarification is required as to whether the Act also empowers the Inspectors to inspect general practitioners' registers.

Many general practitioners have adopted the policy of recording the batch numbers of drugs they personally administer by injection. Shipman did not follow this policy. Furthermore, the controlled drugs registers used by pharmacies do not include a record of batch numbers. In consequence, it is not possible to accurately follow the trail of an ampoule of diamorphine from its purchase by a pharmacy to its administration to a patient, or eventual destruction if not administered. The routine recording of batch numbers would provide the basis for a more satisfactory audit trail for prescribing of controlled injectable drugs, and consideration should be given to promoting such a policy.

# Eight: The pattern of deaths identified from medical certificates of cause of death

## 8.1 Background

In previous Sections of this report, it has been established that:

- the number of deaths among Shipman's patients was higher than among the patients of a group of comparison practitioners (Section Two);

- the numbers could not be explained by the numbers referred to the coroner (Section Six);

- on the evidence of surviving clinical records (Section Four) and cremation forms (Section Five), a substantial proportion of deaths in each year from 1985 share features typical of the murders of which Shipman was convicted.

Various methods may be used in making comparisons between observed and expected deaths. In this Section, information from the MCCDs issued by Shipman and a group of local general practitioners is used to identify the patterns of deaths among his patients between 1974 and 1998. In Section Nine, information is used relating to all deaths among patients registered with Shipman at any time from 1987 to 1998. There are advantages and disadvantages to each method. The use of information from only those MCCDs issued by general practitioners has the advantage of including local data, but lacks the numbers of patients and practitioners that can be included in the analysis in Section Nine. However, although an analysis based on all deaths in the population has the advantage of greater numbers, the comparison is arguably less relevant.

## 8.2 Methods

The data used in this component of the audit were first presented in Section Two (see Tables 2.1 and 2.2). Analyses of these data were undertaken to determine the observed numbers of deaths in comparison with the numbers that would have been expected. The numbers expected were determined from the numbers of deaths among a group of comparison practitioners caring for patients in Hyde or Todmorden during the years in which Shipman worked in those towns (see Section Two). The patients of Shipman and the comparison practitioners were similar socio-economically, as measured by Jarman and Townsend scores (see Section Three). Analyses were undertaken to account for the numbers, age and gender of the patients of Shipman and the comparison practitioners. The analyses also sought to identify from the information recorded on MCCDs the features typical of the convictions throughout the period 1974–1998 (gender, age groups, place of death and certified causes of deaths).

## 8.3 Findings

### 8.3.1 Number of deaths

Shipman certified a higher number of deaths than would be expected. Table 8.1 shows that the numbers were high in comparison with the other practitioners in all years except 1974, 1983, and 1992. The Table includes the rate of deaths per 1000 registered patients, and assumes that the list sizes remained the same during the years before 1987, since accurate data about list size prior to 1987 were not available. However, if the evidence given by Shipman at his trial is correct, his list size was just over 2000 people in 1977, increasing gradually in subsequent years. If this had been the case, the rate of deaths (deaths/1000 registered patients) 1977–1986 among Shipman's patients indicated in the Table would be an underestimate.

The excess number of deaths among Shipman's patients in each year was calculated from the death rates and estimated list size, using the death rate of patients of the comparison practitioners as the expected death rate. In those years in which Shipman worked for only a few months, the observed rate was applied as the annual rate. If we take the year 1979 from Table 8.1 to illustrate the calculation, the number of deaths per 1000 patients of the comparison practitioners was 5.0. Therefore, the expected number among Shipman's patients would have been 5.0 x 2853/1000 = 14.3. The observed number of deaths was 29, and therefore the excess was 14.7. The excess in any year varied from 10 deaths fewer than expected (1977) to 39 more than expected (1997). The total number of excess deaths was 275.3.

The calculations include four years during which Shipman did not work for a full year (1974, 1975, 1977 and 1998), and therefore the excess is likely to be a slight underestimate. The impact of patient socioeconomic factors has not been taken into account, since there were no meaningful differences between the patients of Shipman and the comparison practitioners (see Section Three). However, patient age and sex should be taken into account, and these are addressed in the analyses that follow.

Table 8.1. The numbers of deaths each year, 1973-1998, certified by Shipman and the comparison practitioners, showing the numbers of registered patients and death certification rate per 1000 registered patients. List sizes prior to 1987 are estimates. *applies to part of a year.

| Year | Shipman | | | Comparison practitioners | | | Expected | Difference (observed -expected) |
|---|---|---|---|---|---|---|---|---|
| | Number of deaths | List size | Deaths/ 1000 patients | Number of deaths | Total list size | Deaths/ 1000 patients | | |
| 1973 | | | | 43 | 11000 | 3.9 | | |
| 1974 | 5* | 2444 | 2.0 | 37 | 8556 | 4.3 | 10.5 | -5.5 |
| 1975 | 17* | 2444 | 7.0 | 50 | 8556 | 5.8 | 14.2 | 2.8 |
| 1976 | | | | 46 | 11000 | 4.2 | | |
| 1977 | 4* | 2853 | 1.4 | 41 | 10296 | 4.0 | 11.4 | -7.4 |
| 1978 | 28 | 2853 | 9.8 | 50 | 10296 | 4.9 | 13.8 | 14.2 |
| 1979 | 29 | 2853 | 10.2 | 51 | 10296 | 5.0 | 14.3 | 14.7 |
| 1980 | 22 | 2853 | 7.7 | 41 | 10296 | 4.0 | 11.4 | 10.6 |
| 1981 | 26 | 2853 | 9.1 | 41 | 10296 | 4.0 | 11.4 | 14.6 |
| 1982 | 21 | 2853 | 7.4 | 42 | 10296 | 4.1 | 11.7 | 9.3 |
| 1983 | 15 | 2853 | 5.3 | 68 | 12361 | 5.5 | 15.7 | -0.7 |
| 1984 | 31 | 2853 | 10.9 | 65 | 14419 | 4.5 | 12.8 | 18.2 |
| 1985 | 26 | 2853 | 9.1 | 55 | 14419 | 3.8 | 10.8 | 15.2 |
| 1986 | 15 | 2853 | 5.6 | 51 | 14419 | 3.5 | 9.9 | 5.1 |
| 1987 | 18 | 2853 | 6.3 | 55 | 14419 | 3.8 | 10.8 | 7.2 |
| 1988 | 20 | 2855 | 7.0 | 50 | 14351 | 3.5 | 10.0 | 10.0 |
| 1989 | 17 | 2863 | 5.9 | 44 | 15508 | 2.8 | 8.0 | 9.0 |
| 1990 | 9 | 2860 | 3.1 | 32 | 15030 | 2.1 | 6.0 | 3.0 |
| 1991 | 12 | 2842 | 4.2 | 37 | 16246 | 2.3 | 6.5 | 5.5 |
| 1992 | 7 | 2931 | 2.4 | 46 | 15887 | 2.9 | 8.5 | -1.5 |
| 1993 | 29 | 3115 | 9.3 | 45 | 15567 | 2.9 | 9.0 | 20.0 |
| 1994 | 17 | 3124 | 5.4 | 48 | 15323 | 3.1 | 9.7 | 7.3 |
| 1995 | 39 | 3070 | 12.7 | 30 | 12641 | 2.4 | 7.4 | 31.6 |
| 1996 | 43 | 3038 | 14.2 | 33 | 9654 | 3.4 | 10.3 | 32.7 |
| 1997 | 47 | 3028 | 15.5 | 24 | 9360 | 2.6 | 7.9 | 39.1 |
| 1998 | 24* | 3046 | 7.9 | 11 | 9025 | 1.2 | 3.7 | 20.3 |
| **Total** | 521 | | | 1136 | | | 245.7 | 275.3 |

## 8.3.2. Age

There was a significant difference between patients certified dead by Shipman and the comparison practitioners in the proportions in different age groups (Table 8.2). A higher proportion of Shipman's patients died between the age of 75 and 84 than those of the comparison practitioners. Table 8.3 shows the proportions of deaths in this age group throughout Shipman's career. The higher proportion of deaths in the 75-84 age group among Shipman's patients is evident from 1979, and was consistent throughout all the years Shipman worked in Hyde, except 1978, 1990, 1992 and 1995 (Table 8.3). In Todmorden in 1975, eight (47.1%) of Shipman's deceased patients were aged 65–74, and four (23.5%) 85 or more. In 1978, the respective numbers were 10 (35.7%) and seven (25.0%).

**Table 8.2. Numbers (%) of patients in different age groups.** ($X_6^2 = 14.8$; $p - 0.005$).

| Age Group | Shipman | | Comparison GPs | |
|---|---|---|---|---|
| | N | % | N | % |
| 0–50 | 12 | 2.3 | 36 | 3.1 |
| 51–64 | 44 | 8.4 | 142 | 12.5 |
| 65–74 | 115 | 22.1 | 263 | 23.2 |
| 75–84 | 226 | 43.4 | 393 | 34.6 |
| 85+ | 124 | 23.8 | 302 | 26.6 |
| | 521 | | 1136 | |

**Table 8.3. The number (%) of deaths in patients aged 75–84 for whom Shipman and the comparison practitioners issued MCCDs.**

| Age Group | Shipman | | Comparison GPs | |
|---|---|---|---|---|
| | N | % | N | % |
| 1974 | 0 | 0 | 12 | 32.4 |
| 1975 | 3 | 17.6 | 18 | 36.0 |
| 1976 | – | – | 18 | 39.1 |
| 1977 | 4 | 100 | 15 | 36.6 |
| 1978 | 10 | 35.7 | 22 | 44.0 |
| 1979 | 13 | 44.8 | 17 | 33.3 |
| 1980 | 9 | 40.9 | 11 | 26.8 |
| 1981 | 10 | 38.5 | 12 | 29.3 |
| 1982 | 10 | 47.6 | 13 | 31.0 |
| 1983 | 7 | 46.7 | 23 | 33.8 |
| 1984 | 16 | 51.6 | 27 | 41.5 |
| 1985 | 12 | 46.2 | 20 | 36.4 |
| 1986 | 8 | 53.3 | 18 | 35.3 |
| 1987 | 10 | 55.6 | 27 | 49.1 |
| 1988 | 7 | 35.0 | 17 | 34.0 |
| 1989 | 9 | 52.9 | 15 | 34.1 |
| 1990 | 3 | 33.3 | 14 | 43.8 |
| 1991 | 7 | 58.3 | 11 | 29.7 |
| 1992 | 2 | 28.6 | 14 | 30.4 |
| 1993 | 11 | 37.9 | 9 | 20.0 |
| 1994 | 6 | 35.3 | 12 | 25.0 |
| 1995 | 12 | 30.8 | 13 | 43.3 |
| 1996 | 23 | 53.5 | 7 | 21.2 |
| 1997 | 23 | 48.9 | 9 | 37.5 |
| 1998 | 11 | 45.8 | 4 | 36.4 |

## 8.3.3. Gender

Of the 521 deaths certified by Shipman, 367 (70.4%) were females, but of the 1136 deaths certified by the comparison general practitioners, 608 (53.5%) were females ($X_1^2$ = 42.2; p – 0.000). The proportion of females was higher among deaths certified by Shipman for each year except 1985 and 1995 (Figure 8.1).

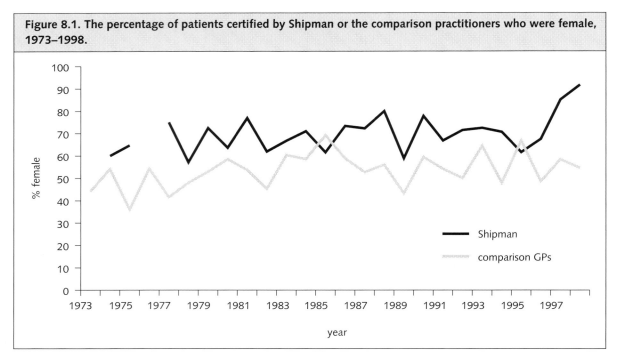

**Figure 8.1. The percentage of patients certified by Shipman or the comparison practitioners who were female, 1973–1998.**

There were differences between Shipman and the comparison practitioners in the numbers of deaths in different age groups in females (Table 8.4).

**Table 8.4 The numbers (%) of females in each age group for whom Shipman or the comparison practitioners issued MCCDs 1973–1998.** *Females* ($X_6^2$ = 22.4; *p* – 0.000), *males* ($X_6^2$ = 8.9; *p* – 0.063).

| Age group | 0–50 | | 51–64 | | 65–74 | | 75–84 | | 85 or above | | Total |
|---|---|---|---|---|---|---|---|---|---|---|---|
| | n | % | n | % | n | % | n | % | n | % | |
| **Females** | | | | | | | | | | | |
| Shipman | 3 | 0.8 | 26 | 7.1 | 74 | 20.2 | 168 | 45.8 | 96 | 26.2 | 367 |
| Comparison GPs | 12 | 2.0 | 44 | 7.2 | 97 | 16.0 | 215 | 35.4 | 240 | 39.5 | 608 |
| **Males** | | | | | | | | | | | |
| Shipman | 9 | 5.8 | 18 | 11.7 | 41 | 26.6 | 58 | 37.7 | 28 | 18.2 | 154 |
| Comparison GPs | 24 | 4.5 | 98 | 18.6 | 166 | 31.4 | 178 | 33.7 | 62 | 11.7 | 528 |

Patients are classified into three age bands by Health Authorities for calculating payments to general practitioners. The age bands are 0-64, 65–74, and 75 and above. Information about general practitioners' lists in this form was available from West Pennine Health Authority from 1991 onwards (Table 3.1). Therefore, it was possible to calculate the numbers of MCCDs issued by Shipman and the comparison practitioners per thousand registered patients in each age/sex group (Tables 8.5 and 8.6). From 1987–1990, data were available about the numbers in each age group, but not gender. Therefore, in calculating death rates, the proportions who were males or females were estimated based on the proportions in 1991. Prior to 1987, no data were available about the numbers of patients, and the numbers as they were in 1987 were used, taking account of the numbers of general practitioners in the comparison group working in each year.

The number of patients registered with the Todmorden practice was assumed to be 11,000. No record of the practice list size in 1973-6 is available, but a general practitioner who was a partner in the practice at that time recalled the list being between 10,000 and 12,000 people. The proportions in different age groups in the practice in 1990 were similar to the proportions registered with the comparison practitioners in Hyde, and it was assumed the list in 1973-76 had the same age/sex distribution (males 75/+ – 2.3%, females 75/+ – 4.3%, females 65–74 – 5.2%, males 65–74 – 4%, males 0-64 – 42.1%, females 0-64 – 42.1%).

Tables 8.5 and 8.6 present the death rates based on these assumptions, and confirm that the death rate was higher among Shipman's male and female patients in the 65–74 and 75 and above age groups. This difference was both more consistent and greater in those aged 75 or above, and particularly among females. One factor that might be argued to explain some of the difference in that some of the comparison practitioners did not work throughout the same period as Shipman. In the years they joined or left their practices, they would be unlikely to have worked complete years. This factor relates to doctor 1 (1996), doctor 4 (1983) and doctor 6 (1982) in Table 2.1. However, the differences in death rates are not particularly marked in these years, and working for only part of a year cannot explain the differences in certain age/sex groups. Furthermore, Shipman himself worked four incomplete years during his career as a general practitioner.

**Table 8.5. The annual numbers of MCCDs issued per 1000 patients in three age groups (0–64, 65–74, 75 and above), in male patients of Shipman and the comparison practitioners.**

| Year | Deaths/1000, males under 65 | | Deaths/1000, 65–74 age group, males | | Deaths/1000, 75 and above, males | |
|------|---------|----------------|---------|----------------|---------|----------------|
| | Shipman | Comparison GPs | Shipman | Comparison GPs | Shipman | Comparison GPs |
| 1973 | | 1.68 | | 13.70 | | 40.16 |
| 1974 | 1.94 | 2.43 | 0 | 8.80 | 0 | 25.77 |
| 1975 | .98 | 1.89 | 20.62 | 35.19 | 52.63 | 67.01 |
| 1976 | | .84 | | 15.98 | | 40.16 |
| 1977 | 0 | 0 | 0 | 21.95 | 14.93 | 64.38 |
| 1978 | .82 | .90 | 63.16 | 19.51 | 74.63 | 60.09 |
| 1979 | 1.64 | 2.02 | 10.53 | 26.83 | 74.63 | 17.17 |
| 1980 | 0 | 1.79 | 42.11 | 17.07 | 59.70 | 8.58 |
| 1981 | 0 | 1.34 | 10.53 | 21.95 | 74.63 | 17.17 |
| 1982 | .82 | 1.57 | 21.05 | 21.95 | 74.63 | 30.04 |
| 1983 | .82 | 1.68 | 10.53 | 4.07 | 44.78 | 57.14 |
| 1984 | 0 | .64 | 21.05 | 20.91 | 104.48 | 33.64 |
| 1985 | 2.45 | .16 | 21.05 | 8.71 | 74.63 | 33.64 |
| 1986 | .82 | .64 | 10.53 | 8.71 | 29.85 | 36.70 |
| 1987 | .82 | .64 | 10.53 | 8.71 | 44.78 | 51.99 |
| 1988 | 0 | 1.12 | 10.53 | 14.06 | 44.78 | 21.94 |
| 1989 | 0 | .90 | 40.40 | 14.35 | 46.15 | 27.03 |
| 1990 | 1.62 | .15 | 0 | 6.36 | 0 | 22.10 |
| 1991 | 1.65 | .58 | 10.87 | 7.54 | 15.63 | 21.22 |
| 1992 | .80 | .89 | 10.31 | 7.70 | 0 | 31.33 |
| 1993 | .75 | .30 | 28.04 | 10.69 | 66.67 | 18.57 |
| 1994 | 2.19 | .76 | 10.31 | 14.79 | 15.63 | 27.10 |
| 1995 | 1.48 | 0 | 34.48 | 5.42 | 156.25 | 20.17 |
| 1996 | 1.49 | .96 | 22.47 | 7.50 | 156.25 | 34.36 |
| 1997 | .75 | .74 | 23.26 | 2.60 | 59.70 | 21.66 |
| 1998 | 0 | 0 | 0 | 2.86 | 31.25 | 14.60 |

**Table 8.6. The annual numbers of MCCDs issued per 1000 patients in three age groups (0–64, 65–74, 75 and above), in female patients of Shipman and the comparison practitioners.**

| Year | Deaths/1000, females under 65 | | Deaths/1000, 65–74 age group, females | | Deaths/1000, 75 and above, females | |
|---|---|---|---|---|---|---|
| | Shipman | Comparison GPs | Shipman | Comparison GPs | Shipman | Comparison GPs |
| 1973 | | .22 | | 3.51 | | 33.54 |
| 1974 | .97 | .86 | 7.87 | 11.31 | 9.62 | 32.35 |
| 1975 | .97 | 1.14 | 47.24 | 4.53 | 38.46 | 32.35 |
| 1976 | | .67 | | 10.54 | | 33.54 |
| 1977 | 0 | .95 | 0 | 7.52 | 24.29 | 20.13 |
| 1978 | 0 | .48 | 32.52 | 7.52 | 99.17 | 40.27 |
| 1979 | 0 | .48 | 32.52 | 7.52 | 140.50 | 46.98 |
| 1980 | 0 | .24 | 0 | 3.76 | 115.70 | 46.98 |
| 1981 | .82 | .48 | 16.26 | 7.52 | 140.50 | 35.79 |
| 1982 | .82 | .71 | 16.26 | 3.76 | 82.64 | 31.32 |
| 1983 | .82 | .40 | 0 | 14.08 | 74.38 | 55.97 |
| 1984 | 2.45 | .34 | 32.52 | 8.04 | 123.97 | 47.92 |
| 1985 | 0 | 1.02 | 48.78 | 8.04 | 82.64 | 41.53 |
| 1986 | .1.63 | .34 | 16.26 | 9.38 | 57.85 | 33.55 |
| 1987 | .0 | .34 | 24.39 | 4.02 | 82.64 | 38.34 |
| 1988 | .82 | .51 | 8.06 | 2.71 | 115.70 | 37.64 |
| 1989 | 0 | 0 | 7.81 | 3.69 | 76.92 | 22.35 |
| 1990 | 1.62 | .49 | 16.95 | 3.67 | 25.86 | 18.73 |
| 1991 | .81 | .60 | 0 | 3.46 | 60.34 | 16.29 |
| 1992 | 0 | .15 | 7.87 | 5.82 | 36.36 | 21.77 |
| 1993 | 1.45 | .16 | 30.53 | 4.61 | 147.06 | 31.87 |
| 1994 | .73 | .33 | 14.93 | 3.50 | 89.11 | 24.66 |
| 1995 | 1.49 | .20 | 75.00 | 4.22 | 123.81 | 25.20 |
| 1996 | 2.26 | 0 | 24.59 | 5.86 | 244.68 | 26.58 |
| 1997 | 3.01 | .27 | 83.33 | 2.03 | 298.85 | 23.76 |
| 1998 | 2.23 | .29 | 61.95 | 2.16 | 155.84 | 7.78 |

## 8.3.4. Place of death

Of those patients certified by Shipman, 75% died at home, compared to 70% of the patients of comparison practitioners (Table 8.7). However, between 1977 and 1983, a greater proportion of deaths certified by the comparison practitioners died at home (Figure 8.3).

**Table 8.7 The numbers (%) of deaths certified by Shipman and the comparison practitioners showing place of death. ($X_4^2 = 22.3$; $p - 0.000$).**

| Place | Shipman | | Comparison Practitioners | | Total | |
|---|---|---|---|---|---|---|
| | n | % | n | % | n | % |
| own home | 391 | 75.0 | 798 | 70.2 | 1189 | 71.8 |
| nursing home | 17 | 3.3 | 51 | 4.5 | 68 | 4.1 |
| residential home | 104 | 20.0 | 244 | 21.5 | 348 | 21.0 |
| practice | 6 | 1.2 | 2 | 0.2 | 8 | 0.5 |
| hospital | 3 | 0.6 | 41 | 3.6 | 44 | 2.7 |
| total | 521 | 100 | 1136 | 100 | 1657 | 100 |

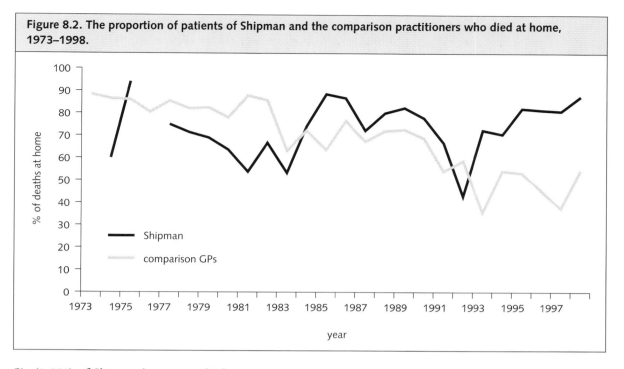

**Figure 8.2. The proportion of patients of Shipman and the comparison practitioners who died at home, 1973–1998.**

Six (1.2%) of Shipman's patients died on practice premises, one in 1989 in the group practice and five in the single-handed practice (one in 1994, two in 1995, one in 1996 and one in 1997). Two (0.2%) of the deaths certified by the comparison practitioners occurred on practice premises.

The finding that between 1977 and 1983, the proportion of patients dying at home was lower among Shipman's patients raises the possibility that at that time he cared for a relatively large number of people living in residential or nursing homes. If this had been the case, a higher rate of death among his elderly patients would have been expected since people in residential or nursing homes would generally have more health problems than those still living in their own homes. It should be noted that of the 102 cases classified as highly suspicious on review of the clinical records (Tables 4.4), only one occurred in a residential home and none in a nursing home.

Tables 8.8 and 8.9 indicate the numbers of MCCDs issued by Shipman and the comparison practitioners for deaths that occurred at home or on practice premises. The data are expressed as numbers of deaths per 1000 registered patients per year, in the six age/sex groups, and the same assumptions described above about list size and proportions in each age/sex group between 1977–1986 have been made. The figures clearly demonstrate an excess of deaths among Shipman's patients in both males and females. The difference is most marked and most consistent among females aged 75 or above. In some years, Shipman had no deaths at home or on practice premises in certain age groups, for example 1992. The total number of deaths in these years was low (see Table 8.1). Shipman did not issue an MCCD for a death occurring at home in 1977.

Table 8.8. Numbers of MCCDs issued per 1000 registered patients in three age groups (0–64, 65–74, 75 and above), males dying at home, patients of Shipman and the comparison practitioners.

| Year | Deaths at home/ 1000, males under 65 | | Deaths/1000, 65–74 age group, males | | Deaths/1000, 75 and above, males | |
|---|---|---|---|---|---|---|
| | Shipman | Comparison GPs | Shipman | Comparison GPs | Shipman | Comparison GPs |
| 1973 | | 1.47 | | 13.70 | | 36.14 |
| 1974 | .97 | 1.89 | 0 | 8.80 | 0 | 25.77 |
| 1975 | .97 | 1.35 | 10.31 | 32.26 | 52.63 | 61.86 |
| 1976 | | .63 | | 13.70 | | 28.11 |
| 1977 | 0 | 0 | 0 | 19.51 | 14.93 | 64.38 |
| 1978 | .82 | .90 | 52.63 | 19.51 | 74.63 | 51.50 |
| 1979 | 1.64 | 2.02 | 10.53 | 26.83 | 44.78 | 12.88 |
| 1980 | 0 | 1.79 | 42.11 | 14.63 | 44.78 | 8.58 |
| 1981 | 0 | 1.34 | 10.53 | 21.95 | 59.70 | 17.17 |
| 1982 | .82 | 1.57 | 21.05 | 21.95 | 74.63 | 25.75 |
| 1983 | .82 | 1.49 | 10.53 | 4.07 | 44.78 | 46.43 |
| 1984 | 0 | .48 | 21.05 | 17.42 | 74.63 | 24.46 |
| 1985 | 2.45 | .16 | 21.05 | 6.97 | 74.63 | 30.58 |
| 1986 | .82 | .64 | 10.53 | 8.71 | 29.85 | 36.70 |
| 1987 | .82 | .64 | 10.53 | 8.71 | 44.78 | 48.93 |
| 1988 | 0 | .96 | 10.53 | 12.30 | 44.78 | 18.81 |
| 1989 | 0 | .75 | 40.40 | 14.35 | 46.15 | 21.62 |
| 1990 | 1.62 | .15 | 0 | 6.36 | 0 | 13.81 |
| 1991 | 1.65 | .58 | 10.87 | 4.52 | 0 | 10.61 |
| 1992 | .80 | .89 | 10.31 | 7.70 | 0 | 13.05 |
| 1993 | .75 | .30 | 18.69 | 4.58 | 50.0 | 7.96 |
| 1994 | 2.19 | .76 | 0 | 8.88 | 15.63 | 10.84 |
| 1995 | 1.48 | 0 | 34.48 | 3.62 | 125.00 | 14.41 |
| 1996 | 1.49 | .96 | 22.47 | 5.00 | 125.00 | 10.31 |
| 1997 | .75 | .74 | 11.63 | 2.60 | 29.85 | 7.22 |
| 1998 | 0 | 0 | 0 | 0 | 31.25 | 10.95 |

Table 8.9. Numbers of MCCDs issued per 1000 registered patients in three age groups (0–64, 65–74, 75 and above), females dying at home, patients of Shipman and the comparison practitioners.

| Year | Deaths at home/ 1000, females under 65 | | Deaths/1000, 65–74 age group, females | | Deaths/1000, 75 and above, females | |
|---|---|---|---|---|---|---|
| | Shipman | Comparison GPs | Shipman | Comparison GPs | Shipman | Comparison GPs |
| 1973 | | .22 | | 1.76 | | 29.35 |
| 1974 | 0 | .57 | 7.87 | 11.31 | 9.62 | 26.95 |
| 1975 | .97 | .86 | 47.24 | 4.52 | 38.46 | 26.95 |
| 1976 | | .67 | | 10.54 | | 25.16 |
| 1977 | 0 | .95 | 0 | 5.64 | 16.53 | 11.19 |
| 1978 | 0 | .48 | 24.39 | 7.65 | 49.59 | 24.60 |
| 1979 | 0 | .48 | 32.52 | 7.52 | 82.64 | 29.08 |
| 1980 | 0 | .24 | 0 | 1.88 | 57.85 | 31.32 |
| 1981 | .82 | .48 | 16.26 | 5.64 | 49.59 | 26.85 |
| 1982 | .82 | .71 | 16.26 | 3.76 | 24.79 | 20.13 |
| 1983 | .82 | .40 | 0 | 10.95 | 16.53 | 20.52 |
| 1984 | 2.45 | .34 | 32.52 | 8.04 | 74.38 | 28.75 |
| 1985 | 0 | .68 | 48.78 | 8.04 | 57.85 | 15.97 |
| 1986 | 1.63 | .34 | 8.13 | 8.04 | 49.59 | 15.97 |
| 1987 | 0 | .34 | 24.39 | 4.02 | 41.32 | 11.18 |
| 1988 | .82 | .51 | 8.06 | 2.71 | 82.64 | 18.00 |
| 1989 | 0 | 0 | 7.81 | 3.69 | 59.83 | 9.78 |
| 1990 | 1.62 | .33 | 8.47 | 2.45 | 17.24 | 11.53 |
| 1991 | .81 | .60 | 0 | 3.46 | 34.48 | 2.51 |
| 1992 | 0 | .15 | 7.87 | 5.82 | 0 | 7.68 |
| 1993 | 1.45 | .16 | 30.53 | 3.46 | 88.24 | 5.31 |
| 1994 | .74 | .33 | 14.93 | 3.50 | 59.41 | 8.22 |
| 1995 | 1.49 | .20 | 66.67 | 2.81 | 104.76 | 9.45 |
| 1996 | 1.50 | 0 | 24.59 | 5.86 | 212.77 | 6.13 |
| 1997 | 3.01 | .27 | 75.00 | 2.03 | 252.87 | 3.96 |
| 1998 | 2.23 | .29 | 53.10 | 2.16 | 129.87 | 3.89 |

## 8.3.5. The effect of different assumptions about patient lists 1977–1986

The foregoing calculations of death rates for the years 1977–1986 rest upon an assumption about the numbers of patients registered with Shipman during this period. It has been assumed that the total numbers and proportions in different age/sex groups were more or less constant. The age and sex distribution of the population in Hyde was very similar in 1981 and 1997 (Table 8.10) and it is therefore reasonable to assume that the population registered with a group of practitioners such as the comparison practitioners would likewise remain similar. However, the composition of the population registered with an individual practitioner is at greater risk of being less representative since the total number of people is smaller and local circumstances may be more influential.

In order to test for the effect of different assumptions about the registered list of patients on the estimated death rates, two additional analyses were undertaken for the years 1977–1986. In the first scenario, it was assumed that Shipman's list size in 1977 was 2000, as he had claimed at the trial. The list was assumed to gradually increase to its actual level of 2853 in 1987. The proportions in different age/sex bands were assumed to be those of the general population of Hyde in 1981 (females aged above 75 – 3.8% of total population, males above 75 – 1.7%, females 65 to 74 – 5.5% and males – 4.1%).

The deaths per thousand patients in different age and sex groups calculated based on the assumptions of the first scenario are shown in Table 8.11. As a consequence of the smaller total list size, and the reduction in the numbers aged 75 and above, the death rates in this age group have risen.

### Table 8.10. Numbers (%) of people in Hyde in different age and sex groups in the 1981 Census and in the 1997 Local Population Survey.

| Age Group | 1997 survey | | | | | 1981 census | | | | |
| | Males | | Females | | Total | Males | | Females | | Total |
| | n | % | n | % | n | n | % | n | % | n |
|---|---|---|---|---|---|---|---|---|---|---|
| 0-64 | 16025 | 50.3 | 15855 | 49.7 | 31880 | 15315 | 50.7 | 14908 | 49.3 | 30223 |
| 65–74 | 1425 | 41.2 | 2035 | 58.8 | 3460 | 1452 | 42.5 | 1966 | 57.5 | 3418 |
| 75 or more | 505 | 30.9 | 1130 | 69.1 | 1635 | 602 | 30.7 | 1362 | 69.3 | 1964 |
| totals | 17955 | | 19020 | | 36975 | 17369 | | 18236 | | 35605 |

### Table 8.11. MCCDs issued per 1000 registered patients of Shipman, 1977–1986, assuming that Shipman's patient list in 1977 was 2000, gradually increasing to 2853 by 1987, and that the percentages of patients in different age groups matched the 1981 Census. The deaths are those occurring at home or on practice premises, with MCCDs issued by general practitioners.

| Rate/1000 registered patients | Males <65 | Males 65–74 | Males 75+ | Females <65 | Females 65–74 | Females 75+ |
|---|---|---|---|---|---|---|
| year | | | | | | |
| 1977 | | | | | | |
| 1978 | 1.16 | 60.98 | 147.06 | | 27.27 | 77.92 |
| 1979 | 2.27 | 11.90 | 85.71 | | 35.40 | 126.58 |
| 1980 | | 45.45 | 83.33 | | | 85.37 |
| 1981 | | 10.87 | 105.26 | 1.06 | 16.13 | 69.77 |
| 1982 | .99 | 20.83 | 125.00 | 1.02 | 15.38 | 33.33 |
| 1983 | .95 | 10.00 | 73.17 | .98 | | 21.28 |
| 1984 | | 19.23 | 116.28 | 2.81 | 28.37 | 91.84 |
| 1985 | 2.63 | 18.52 | 111.11 | | 41.10 | 69.31 |
| 1986 | .85 | 8.93 | 43.48 | 1.74 | 6.58 | 57.14 |

In the second scenario, it was assumed that Shipman's list of patients in 1977 was as large as at any time from 1977–1998. Since it reached 3124 in 1994, a list size of 3125 was applied for 1977. Furthermore, it was assumed that the proportions in the older age groups were higher, and that they declined gradually to the levels of 1987 (Table 8.12).

| Table 8.12 The percentages of Shipman's registered patient population assumed to be in different age/sex groups for the analysis reported in Table 8.13. | | | | |
|---|---|---|---|---|
| | 1977 – 1981 | | 1982 – 1986 | |
| | Males | females | males | females |
| 0–64 | 39.5 | 39.5 | 40.6 | 40.6 |
| 65–74 | 5 | 6.0 | 4.3 | 5.5 |
| 75 + | 4 | 6.0 | 3.5 | 5.5 |

| Table 8.13. MCCDs relating to deaths at home or on practice permises issued per 1000 registered patients of Shipman, 1977–1986, assuming that Shipman's patient list in 1977 was 3125, gradually falling to 2853 by 1987, and that the percentages of patients in the age groups 65–74 and 75 and over were greater than in the 1981 Census (see Table 8.12). | | | | | | |
|---|---|---|---|---|---|---|
| Rate/1000 registered patients | Males <65 | Males 65–74 | Males 75+ | Females <65 | Females 65–74 | Females 75+ |
| **year** | | | | | | |
| 1977 | | | | | | |
| 1978 | .81 | 32.05 | 40.00 | | 15.96 | 31.91 |
| 1979 | 1.62 | 6.42 | 24.00 | | 21.28 | 53.19 |
| 1980 | | 25.82 | 24.19 | | | 37.63 |
| 1981 | | 6.49 | 32.26 | .82 | 10.81 | 32.43 |
| 1982 | .80 | 15.15 | 46.30 | .80 | 11.83 | 17.75 |
| 1983 | .81 | 7.63 | 28.04 | .81 | | 11.90 |
| 1984 | | 15.38 | 47.17 | 2.44 | 24.10 | 54.22 |
| 1985 | 2.46 | 15.50 | 47.62 | | 36.36 | 42.42 |
| 1986 | .84 | 7.94 | 19.42 | 1.68 | 6.17 | 37.04 |

The findings calculated using the assumptions of the second scenario are shown in Table 8.13. In many of the years, the death rates in the older age groups were higher than those of the comparison practitioners despite the assumed larger total list size and greater proportions of older people (for comparison practitioners' rates, see Tables 8.8 and 8.9).

The scenarios presented in Tables 8.11 and 8.13 are based on assumptions deliberately chosen because they represent the extremes of what might have been the list of patients registered with Shipman from 1977. In view of the tendency of patient lists in Hyde to be relatively large, a list size of 2000 that only slowly increased from 1977 is unlikely. On the other hand, a list size of 3125 with a high proportion of elderly patients would have been equally unlikely. If the observed death rates among Shipman's patients, calculated on both these extreme assumptions, are higher than the rate of the comparison practitioners, a high degree of confidence can be placed on the conclusion that the numbers of MCCDs issued by Shipman, even in the early years in his career (1978–86), were higher than would have been expected.

The relationship between the rates based on the two scenarios of Shipman's list and the rates for the comparison practitioners are shown in Figures 8.3-8.6. The 0–64 year age groups are not included since there were no differences between Shipman and the comparison practitioners in these groups. Among both males and females aged 75 and above, there were clear differences between both list scenarios and the comparison practitioners (Figures 8.4 and 8.6). The difference was evident for all years except 1983 and, in males, 1978. There were also differences among females aged 65-74 (Figure 8.5), although in some years Shipman did not issue any MCCDs for deaths at home in this group. Among males aged 65–74 (Figure 8.4), the difference was less consistent.

It is possible, therefore, to conclude that from 1978 to 1986, Shipman did issue an excess of MCCDs for deaths occurring at home, among both male and female patients aged 75 or above. The rates among females aged 65–74 were also high, although the rates among males in that age group were less clearly raised.

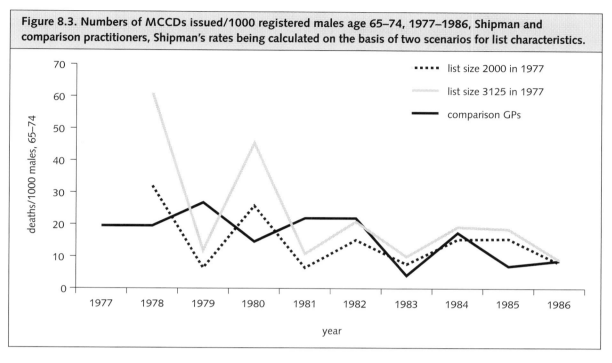

**Figure 8.3. Numbers of MCCDs issued/1000 registered males age 65–74, 1977–1986, Shipman and comparison practitioners, Shipman's rates being calculated on the basis of two scenarios for list characteristics.**

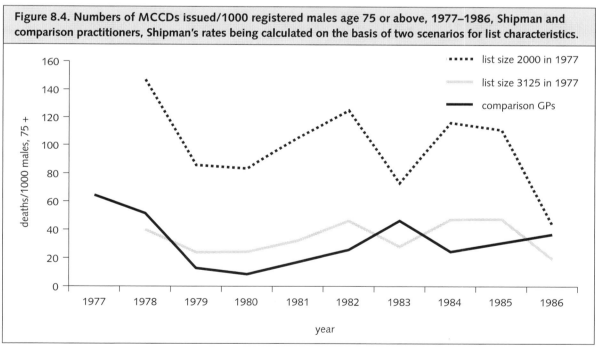

**Figure 8.4. Numbers of MCCDs issued/1000 registered males age 75 or above, 1977–1986, Shipman and comparison practitioners, Shipman's rates being calculated on the basis of two scenarios for list characteristics.**

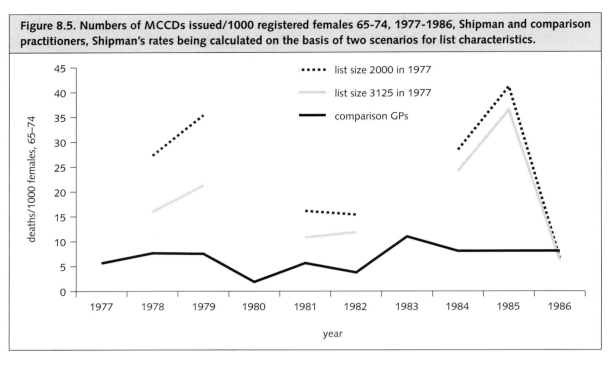

Figure 8.5. Numbers of MCCDs issued/1000 registered females 65-74, 1977-1986, Shipman and comparison practitioners, Shipman's rates being calculated on the basis of two scenarios for list characteristics.

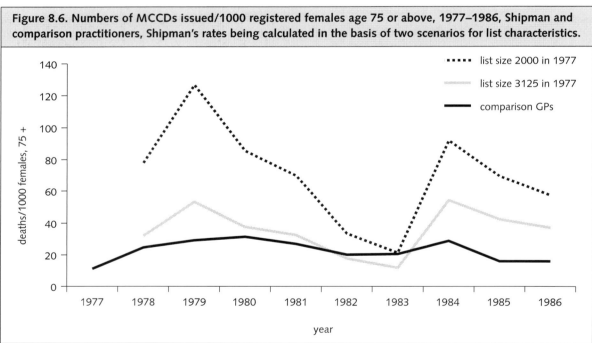

Figure 8.6. Numbers of MCCDs issued/1000 registered females age 75 or above, 1977–1986, Shipman and comparison practitioners, Shipman's rates being calculated in the basis of two scenarios for list characteristics.

## 8.3.6. Excess numbers of deaths in different age/sex groups

Having established that different list scenarios are unlikely to explain the differences between the death rates of the patients of Shipman and the comparison practitioners, an analysis was undertaken to determine the numbers of deaths in excess of those expected. The calculations were repeated for each age/sex group in order to take into account differences between Shipman and the comparison practitioners in the proportions of patients in each group. Since almost all deaths giving rise to concern on review of records or cremation forms had occurred in the patient's home or in the practice, separate analyses were undertaken for all MCCDs and those for deaths at home or in practices only.

The findings are presented in Tables 8.15 - 8.26. Each Table includes the numbers of patients in the relevant age group registered or assumed to be registered with Shipman and the comparison practitioners, the numbers of deaths, the death rate per thousand patients, the numbers of deaths that would have been expected among Shipman's patients, and the difference between the observed and expected numbers of deaths. The list size assumptions are those in the analysis reported in Table 8.1, and lie between the two scenarios reported above (Section 8.3.5). The death rate per thousand patients was calculated as described previously. The expected number of deaths was calculated by multiplying the death rate per thousand patients of the comparison group by Shipman's number of patients, and dividing by 1000.

**Table 8.15. The excess number of deaths per year among Shipman's patients, males aged under 65 years. The figures include all MCCDs issued, irrespective of place of death.**

| Year | Number of males aged under 65 | | Number of deaths | | Deaths/s 1000 pt | | Expected | Difference |
|---|---|---|---|---|---|---|---|---|
| | Shipman | Comp. GPs | Shipman | Comp. GPs | Shipman | Comp. GPs | | |
| 1973 | | 4770 | | 8 | | 1.68 | – | |
| 1974 | 1029 | 3710 | 2 | 9 | 1.94 | 2.43 | 2.50 | -0.5 |
| 1975 | 1029 | 3710 | 1 | 7 | 0.98 | 1.89 | 1.94 | -0.94 |
| 1976 | | 4770 | | 4 | | .84 | | |
| 1977 | 1223 | 4465 | 0 | 0 | 0 | 0 | 0 | 0 |
| 1978 | 1223 | 4465 | 1 | 4 | .82 | .90 | 1.10 | -0.10 |
| 1979 | 1223 | 4465 | 2 | 9 | 1.64 | 2.02 | 2.47 | -0.47 |
| 1980 | 1223 | 4465 | 0 | 8 | 0 | 1.79 | 2.19 | -2.19 |
| 1981 | 1223 | 4465 | 0 | 6 | 0 | 1.34 | 1.64 | -1.64 |
| 1982 | 1223 | 4465 | 1 | 7 | .82 | 1.57 | 1.92 | -.92 |
| 1983 | 1223 | 5360 | 1 | 9 | .82 | 1.68 | 2.05 | -1.05 |
| 1984 | 1223 | 6255 | 0 | 4 | 0 | .64 | 0.78 | -.78 |
| 1985 | 1223 | 6255 | 3 | 1 | 2.45 | .16 | 0.20 | 2.8 |
| 1986 | 1223 | 6255 | 1 | 4 | .82 | .64 | 0.78 | 0.22 |
| 1987 | 1223 | 6255 | 1 | 4 | .82 | .64 | 0.78 | 0.22 |
| 1988 | 1224 | 6239 | 0 | 7 | 0 | 1.12 | 1.37 | -1.37 |
| 1989 | 1227 | 6685 | 0 | 6 | 0 | .90 | 1.10 | -1.10 |
| 1990 | 1235 | 6459 | 2 | 1 | 1.62 | .15 | 0.19 | 1.81 |
| 1991 | 1215 | 6927 | 2 | 4 | 1.65 | .58 | 0.70 | 1.30 |
| 1992 | 1254 | 6772 | 1 | 6 | .80 | .89 | 1.12 | -0.12 |
| 1993 | 1340 | 6646 | 1 | 2 | .75 | .30 | 0.40 | 0.60 |
| 1994 | 1368 | 6554 | 3 | 5 | 2.19 | .76 | 1.04 | 1.96 |
| 1995 | 1353 | 5413 | 2 | 0 | 1.48 | 0 | 0 | 2.0 |
| 1996 | 1340 | 4185 | 2 | 4 | 1.49 | .96 | 1.29 | 0.71 |
| 1997 | 1339 | 4040 | 1 | 3 | .75 | .74 | 0.99 | 0.01 |
| 1998 | 1348 | 3925 | 0 | 0 | | | | |
| total | | | 27 observed | 122 | | | 26.55 expected | 0.45 difference |

**Table 8.16. The excess number of deaths per year among Shipman's patients, females aged under 65 years. The figures include all MCCDs issued, irrespective of place of death.**

| Year | Number of females <65 | | Number of deaths | | Deaths/s 1000 pt | | Expected | Difference |
|---|---|---|---|---|---|---|---|---|
| | Shipman | Comp. GPs | Shipman | Comp. GPs | Shipman | Comp. GPs | | |
| 1973 | | 4492 | | 1 | | 0.22 | - | |
| 1974 | 1030 | 3494 | 1 | 3 | 0.97 | 0.86 | .89 | 0.11 |
| 1975 | 1030 | 3494 | 1 | 4 | 0.97 | 1.14 | 1.17 | -0.17 |
| 1976 | | 4492 | | 3 | | 0.67 | | |
| 1977 | 1224 | 4204 | 0 | 4 | 0 | 0.95 | 1.16 | -1.16 |
| 1978 | 1224 | 4204 | 0 | 2 | 0 | 0.48 | 0.59 | -0.59 |
| 1979 | 1224 | 4204 | 0 | 2 | 0 | 0.48 | 0.59 | -0.59 |
| 1980 | 1224 | 4204 | 0 | 1 | 0 | 0.24 | 0.29 | -0.29 |
| 1981 | 1224 | 4204 | 1 | 2 | 0.82 | 0.48 | 0.59 | 0.23 |
| 1982 | 1224 | 4204 | 1 | 3 | 0.82 | 0.71 | 0.87 | 0.13 |
| 1983 | 1224 | 5048 | 1 | 2 | 0.82 | 0.40 | 0.49 | 0.51 |
| 1984 | 1224 | 5891 | 3 | 2 | 2.45 | 0.34 | 0.42 | 2.58 |
| 1985 | 1224 | 5891 | 0 | 6 | 0 | 1.02 | 1.25 | -1.25 |
| 1986 | 1224 | 5891 | 2 | 2 | 1.63 | 0.34 | 0.42 | 1.58 |
| 1987 | 1224 | 5891 | 0 | 2 | 0 | 0.34 | 0.42 | -0.42 |
| 1988 | 1224 | 5875 | 1 | 3 | 0.82 | 0.51 | 0.62 | 0.38 |
| 1989 | 1227 | 6296 | 0 | 0 | 0 | 0 | 0 | 0 |
| 1990 | 1236 | 6082 | 2 | 3 | 1.62 | 0.49 | 0.60 | 1.40 |
| 1991 | 1240 | 6613 | 1 | 4 | 0.81 | 0.60 | 0.74 | 0.26 |
| 1992 | 1280 | 6479 | 0 | 1 | 0 | 0.15 | 0.19 | -0.19 |
| 1993 | 1375 | 6268 | 2 | 1 | 1.45 | 0.16 | 0.22 | 1.78 |
| 1994 | 1360 | 6138 | 1 | 2 | 0.73 | 0.33 | 0.45 | 0.55 |
| 1995 | 1341 | 4982 | 2 | 1 | 1.49 | 0.20 | 0.27 | 1.73 |
| 1996 | 1329 | 3807 | 3 | 0 | 2.26 | 0 | 0 | 3.0 |
| 1997 | 1329 | 3661 | 4 | 1 | 3.01 | 0.27 | 0.36 | 3.64 |
| 1998 | 1345 | 3499 | 3 | 1 | 2.23 | 0.29 | 0.39 | 2.61 |
| total | | | 29 observed | 56 | | | 12.99 expected | 16.01 difference |

| Table 8.17. The excess number of deaths per year among Shipman's patients, males aged 65–74 years. The figures include all MCCDs issued, irrespective of place of death. | | | | | | | |
|---|---|---|---|---|---|---|---|
| Year | Number of males 65–74 | | Number of deaths | | Deaths/s 1000 pt | | Expected | Difference |
| | Shipman | Comp. GPs | Shipman | Comp. GPs | Shipman | Comp. GPs | | |
| 1973 | | 438 | | 6 | | 13.70 | | |
| 1974 | 97 | 341 | 0 | 3 | 0 | 8.80 | 0.85 | -0.85 |
| 1975 | 97 | 341 | 2 | 12 | 20.62 | 35.19 | 3.41 | -1.41 |
| 1976 | | 438 | | 7 | | 15.98 | | |
| 1977 | 95 | 410 | 0 | 9 | 0 | 21.95 | 2.08 | -2.08 |
| 1978 | 95 | 410 | 6 | 8 | 63.16 | 19.51 | 1.85 | 4.15 |
| 1979 | 95 | 410 | 1 | 11 | 10.53 | 26.83 | 2.55 | -1.55 |
| 1980 | 95 | 410 | 4 | 7 | 42.11 | 17.07 | 1.62 | 2.38 |
| 1981 | 95 | 410 | 1 | 9 | 10.53 | 21.95 | 2.09 | -1.09 |
| 1982 | 95 | 410 | 2 | 9 | 21.05 | 21.95 | 2.09 | -0.09 |
| 1983 | 95 | 492 | 1 | 2 | 10.53 | 4.07 | 0.39 | 0.61 |
| 1984 | 95 | 574 | 2 | 12 | 21.05 | 20.91 | 1.99 | 0.01 |
| 1985 | 95 | 574 | 2 | 5 | 21.05 | 8.71 | 0.83 | 1.17 |
| 1986 | 95 | 574 | 1 | 5 | 10.53 | 8.71 | 0.83 | 0.17 |
| 1987 | 95 | 574 | 1 | 5 | 10.53 | 8.71 | 0.83 | 0.17 |
| 1988 | 95 | 569 | 1 | 8 | 10.53 | 14.06 | 1.34 | -0.34 |
| 1989 | 99 | 627 | 4 | 9 | 40.40 | 14.35 | 1.42 | 2.58 |
| 1990 | 91 | 629 | 0 | 4 | 0 | 6.36 | 0.58 | -0.58 |
| 1991 | 92 | 663 | 1 | 5 | 10.87 | 7.54 | 0.69 | 0.31 |
| 1992 | 97 | 649 | 1 | 5 | 10.31 | 7.70 | 0.75 | 0.25 |
| 1993 | 107 | 655 | 3 | 7 | 28.04 | 10.69 | 1.14 | 1.86 |
| 1994 | 97 | 676 | 1 | 10 | 10.31 | 14.79 | 1.43 | -0.43 |
| 1995 | 87 | 553 | 3 | 3 | 34.48 | 5.42 | 0.47 | 2.53 |
| 1996 | 89 | 400 | 2 | 3 | 22.47 | 7.50 | 0.67 | 1.33 |
| 1997 | 86 | 384 | 2 | 1 | 23.26 | 2.60 | 0.22 | 1.78 |
| 1998 | 99 | 350 | 0 | 1 | 0 | 2.86 | 0.28 | -0.28 |
| total | | | 41 observed | 166 | | | 30.4 expected | 10.60 difference |

| Year | Number of females 65–74 | | Number of deaths | | Deaths/s 1000 pt | | Expected | Difference |
|---|---|---|---|---|---|---|---|---|
| | Shipman | Comp. GPs | Shipman | Comp. GPs | Shipman | Comp. GPs | | |
| 1973 | | 569 | | 2 | | 3.51 | - | |
| 1974 | 127 | 442 | 1 | 5 | 7.87 | 11.31 | 1.44 | -0.44 |
| 1975 | 127 | 442 | 6 | 2 | 47.24 | 4.53 | 0.58 | 5.42 |
| 1976 | | 569 | | 6 | | 10.54 | | |
| 1977 | 123 | 532 | 0 | 4 | 0 | 7.52 | 0.92 | -0.92 |
| 1978 | 123 | 532 | 4 | 4 | 32.52 | 7.52 | 0.92 | 3.08 |
| 1979 | 123 | 532 | 4 | 4 | 32.52 | 7.52 | 0.92 | 3.08 |
| 1980 | 123 | 532 | 0 | 2 | 0 | 3.76 | 0.46 | -0.46 |
| 1981 | 123 | 532 | 2 | 4 | 16.26 | 7.52 | 0.92 | 1.08 |
| 1982 | 123 | 532 | 2 | 2 | 16.26 | 3.76 | 0.46 | 1.54 |
| 1983 | 123 | 639 | 0 | 9 | 0 | 14.08 | 1.73 | -1.73 |
| 1984 | 123 | 746 | 4 | 6 | 32.52 | 8.04 | 0.99 | 3.01 |
| 1985 | 123 | 746 | 6 | 6 | 48.78 | 8.04 | 0.99 | 5.01 |
| 1986 | 123 | 746 | 2 | 7 | 16.26 | 9.38 | 1.15 | 0.85 |
| 1987 | 123 | 746 | 3 | 3 | 24.39 | 4.02 | 0.49 | 2.51 |
| 1988 | 124 | 738 | 1 | 2 | 8.06 | 2.71 | 0.34 | 0.66 |
| 1989 | 128 | 814 | 1 | 3 | 7.81 | 3.69 | 0.47 | 0.53 |
| 1990 | 118 | 817 | 2 | 3 | 16.95 | 3.67 | 0.43 | 1.57 |
| 1991 | 115 | 868 | 0 | 3 | 0 | 3.46 | 0.40 | -0.40 |
| 1992 | 127 | 859 | 1 | 5 | 7.87 | 5.82 | 0.74 | 0.26 |
| 1993 | 131 | 868 | 4 | 4 | 30.53 | 4.61 | 0.60 | 3.40 |
| 1994 | 134 | 856 | 2 | 3 | 14.93 | 3.50 | 0.47 | 1.53 |
| 1995 | 120 | 711 | 9 | 3 | 75.00 | 4.22 | 0.51 | 8.49 |
| 1996 | 122 | 512 | 3 | 3 | 24.59 | 5.86 | 0.71 | 2.29 |
| 1997 | 120 | 493 | 10 | 1 | 83.33 | 2.03 | 0.24 | 9.76 |
| 1998 | 113 | 463 | 7 | 1 | 61.95 | 2.16 | 0.24 | 6.76 |
| total | | | 74 observed | 97 | | | 17.12 expected | 56.88 difference |

Table 8.18. The excess number of deaths per year among Shipman's patients, females aged 65–74 years. The figures include all MCCDs issued, irrespective of place of death.

Table 8.19. The excess number of deaths per year among Shipman's patients, males aged 75 years and above. The figures include all MCCDs issued, irrespective of place of death.

| Year | Number of males 75/+ | | Number of deaths | | Deaths/s 1000 pt | | Expected | Difference |
|------|---------|-----------|---------|-----------|---------|-----------|----------|------------|
|      | Shipman | Comp. GPs | Shipman | Comp. GPs | Shipman | Comp. GPs |          |            |
| 1973 |         | 249       |         | 10        |         | 40.16     |          |            |
| 1974 | 57      | 194       | 0       | 5         | 0       | 25.77     | 1.47     | -1.47      |
| 1975 | 57      | 194       | 3       | 13        | 52.63   | 67.01     | 3.82     | -0.82      |
| 1976 |         | 249       |         | 10        |         | 40.16     |          |            |
| 1977 | 67      | 233       | 1       | 15        | 14.93   | 64.38     | 4.31     | -3.31      |
| 1978 | 67      | 233       | 5       | 14        | 74.63   | 60.09     | 4.03     | 0.97       |
| 1979 | 67      | 233       | 5       | 4         | 74.63   | 17.17     | 1.15     | 3.85       |
| 1980 | 67      | 233       | 4       | 2         | 59.70   | 8.58      | 0.57     | 3.43       |
| 1981 | 67      | 233       | 5       | 4         | 74.63   | 17.17     | 1.15     | 3.85       |
| 1982 | 67      | 233       | 5       | 7         | 74.63   | 30.04     | 2.01     | 2.99       |
| 1983 | 67      | 280       | 3       | 16        | 44.78   | 57.14     | 3.83     | -0.83      |
| 1984 | 67      | 327       | 7       | 11        | 104.48  | 33.64     | 2.25     | 4.75       |
| 1985 | 67      | 327       | 5       | 11        | 74.63   | 33.64     | 2.25     | 2.75       |
| 1986 | 67      | 327       | 2       | 12        | 29.85   | 36.70     | 2.46     | -0.46      |
| 1987 | 67      | 327       | 3       | 17        | 44.78   | 51.99     | 3.48     | -0.48      |
| 1988 | 67      | 319       | 3       | 7         | 44.78   | 21.94     | 1.47     | 1.53       |
| 1989 | 65      | 370       | 3       | 10        | 46.15   | 27.03     | 1.76     | 1.24       |
| 1990 | 64      | 362       | 0       | 8         | 0       | 22.10     | 1.41     | -1.41      |
| 1991 | 64      | 377       | 1       | 8         | 15.63   | 21.22     | 1.36     | -0.36      |
| 1992 | 63      | 383       | 0       | 12        | 0       | 31.33     | 1.97     | -1.97      |
| 1993 | 60      | 377       | 4       | 7         | 66.67   | 18.57     | 1.11     | 2.89       |
| 1994 | 64      | 369       | 1       | 10        | 15.63   | 27.10     | 1.73     | -0.73      |
| 1995 | 64      | 347       | 10      | 7         | 156.25  | 20.17     | 1.29     | 8.71       |
| 1996 | 64      | 291       | 10      | 10        | 156.25  | 34.36     | 2.20     | 7.80       |
| 1997 | 67      | 277       | 4       | 6         | 59.70   | 21.66     | 1.45     | 2.55       |
| 1998 | 64      | 274       | 2       | 4         | 31.25   | 14.60     | 0.93     | 1.07       |
| total |        |           | 86 observed | 240 |     |           | 49.46 expected | 36.54 difference |

Table 8.20. The excess number of deaths per year among Shipman's patients, females aged 75 years or above. The figures include all MCCDs issued, irrespective of place of death.

| Year | Number of females 75/+ | | Number of deaths | | Deaths/s 1000 pt | | Expected | Difference |
|------|---------|------------|---------|------------|---------|------------|----------|------------|
| | Shipman | Comp. GPs | Shipman | Comp. GPs | Shipman | Comp. GPs | | |
| 1973 | | 477 | | 16 | | 33.54 | | |
| 1974 | 104 | 371 | 1 | 12 | 9.62 | 32.35 | 3.36 | -2.36 |
| 1975 | 104 | 371 | 4 | 12 | 38.46 | 32.35 | 3.36 | 0.64 |
| 1976 | | 477 | | 16 | | 33.54 | | |
| 1977 | 121 | 447 | 3 | 9 | 24.29 | 20.13 | 2.44 | 0.56 |
| 1978 | 121 | 447 | 12 | 18 | 99.17 | 40.27 | 4.87 | 7.13 |
| 1979 | 121 | 447 | 17 | 21 | 140.50 | 46.98 | 5.68 | 11.32 |
| 1980 | 121 | 447 | 14 | 21 | 115.70 | 46.98 | 5.68 | 8.32 |
| 1981 | 121 | 447 | 17 | 16 | 140.50 | 35.79 | 4.33 | 12.67 |
| 1982 | 121 | 447 | 10 | 14 | 82.64 | 31.32 | 3.79 | 6.21 |
| 1983 | 121 | 536 | 9 | 30 | 74.38 | 55.97 | 6.77 | 2.23 |
| 1984 | 121 | 626 | 15 | 30 | 123.97 | 47.92 | 5.80 | 9.20 |
| 1985 | 121 | 626 | 10 | 26 | 82.64 | 41.53 | 5.03 | 4.97 |
| 1986 | 121 | 626 | 7 | 21 | 57.85 | 33.55 | 4.06 | 2.94 |
| 1987 | 121 | 626 | 10 | 24 | 82.64 | 38.34 | 4.64 | 5.36 |
| 1988 | 121 | 611 | 14 | 23 | 115.70 | 37.64 | 4.55 | 9.45 |
| 1989 | 117 | 716 | 9 | 16 | 76.93 | 22.35 | 2.61 | 6.39 |
| 1990 | 116 | 694 | 3 | 13 | 25.86 | 18.73 | 2.17 | 0.83 |
| 1991 | 116 | 798 | 7 | 13 | 60.34 | 16.29 | 1.89 | 5.11 |
| 1992 | 110 | 781 | 4 | 17 | 36.36 | 21.77 | 2.39 | 1.61 |
| 1993 | 102 | 753 | 15 | 24 | 147.06 | 31.87 | 3.25 | 11.75 |
| 1994 | 101 | 730 | 9 | 18 | 89.11 | 24.66 | 2.49 | 6.51 |
| 1995 | 105 | 635 | 13 | 16 | 123.81 | 25.20 | 2.65 | 10.35 |
| 1996 | 94 | 489 | 23 | 13 | 244.68 | 25.58 | 2.40 | 20.60 |
| 1997 | 87 | 505 | 26 | 12 | 298.85 | 23.76 | 2.07 | 23.93 |
| 1998 | 77 | 514 | 12 | 4 | 155.84 | 7.78 | 0.60 | 11.4 |
| total | | | 264 observed | 455 | | | 86.88 expected | 177.12 difference |

| Year | Number of males <65 | | Number of deaths | | Deaths/s 1000 pt | | Expected | Difference |
|------|------|------|------|------|------|------|------|------|
| | Shipman | Comp. GPs | Shipman | Comp. GPs | Shipman | Comp. GPs | | |
| 1973 | | 4770 | | 7 | | 1.47 | | |
| 1974 | 1029 | 3710 | 1 | 7 | 0.97 | 1.89 | 1.94 | -0.94 |
| 1975 | 1029 | 3710 | 1 | 5 | 0.97 | 1.35 | 1.39 | -.39 |
| 1976 | | 4770 | | 3 | | 0.63 | | |
| 1977 | 1223 | 4465 | 0 | 0 | 0 | 0 | 0 | 0 |
| 1978 | 1223 | 4465 | 1 | 4 | 0.82 | 0.90 | 1.10 | -0.10 |
| 1979 | 1223 | 4465 | 2 | 9 | 1.64 | 2.02 | 2.47 | -0.47 |
| 1980 | 1223 | 4465 | 0 | 8 | 0 | 1.79 | 2.19 | -2.19 |
| 1981 | 1223 | 4465 | 0 | 6 | 0 | 1.34 | 1.64 | -1.64 |
| 1982 | 1223 | 4465 | 1 | 7 | 0.82 | 1.57 | 1.92 | -0.92 |
| 1983 | 1223 | 5360 | 1 | 8 | 0.82 | 1.49 | 1.82 | -0.82 |
| 1984 | 1223 | 6255 | 0 | 3 | 0 | 0.48 | 0.59 | -0.59 |
| 1985 | 1223 | 6255 | 3 | 1 | 2.45 | 0.16 | 0.20 | 2.80 |
| 1986 | 1223 | 6255 | 1 | 4 | 0.82 | 0.64 | 0.78 | 0.22 |
| 1987 | 1223 | 6255 | 1 | 4 | 0.82 | 0.64 | 0.78 | 0.22 |
| 1988 | 1224 | 6239 | 0 | 6 | 0 | 0.96 | 1.18 | -1.18 |
| 1989 | 1227 | 6685 | 0 | 5 | 0 | 0.75 | 0.92 | -0.92 |
| 1990 | 1235 | 6459 | 2 | 1 | 1.62 | 0.15 | 0.19 | 1.81 |
| 1991 | 1215 | 6927 | 2 | 4 | 1.65 | 0.58 | 0.70 | 1.30 |
| 1992 | 1254 | 6772 | 1 | 6 | 0.80 | 0.89 | 1.12 | -0.12 |
| 1993 | 1340 | 6646 | 1 | 2 | 0.75 | 0.30 | 0.40 | 0.60 |
| 1994 | 1368 | 6554 | 3 | 5 | 2.19 | 0.76 | 1.04 | 1.96 |
| 1995 | 1353 | 5413 | 2 | 0 | 1.48 | 0 | 0 | 2.00 |
| 1996 | 1340 | 4185 | 1 | 4 | 0.75 | 0.96 | 1.29 | -0.29 |
| 1997 | 1339 | 4040 | 1 | 3 | 0.75 | 0.74 | 0.99 | 0.01 |
| 1998 | 1348 | 3925 | 0 | 0 | 0 | 0 | 0 | 0 |
| total | | | 25 observed | 112 | | | 24.65 expected | 0.35 difference |

Table 8.21. The excess number of deaths per year among Shipman's patients, males aged under 65 years. The figures include only MCCDs issued for deaths occurring in the patient's home or on practice premises.

Table 8.22. The excess number of deaths per year among Shipman's patients, females aged under 65 years. The figures include only MCCDs issued for deaths occurring in the patient's home or on practice premises.

| Year | Number of females <65 Shipman | Comp. GPs | Number of deaths Shipman | Comp. GPs | Deaths/s 1000 pt Shipman | Comp. GPs | Expected | Difference |
|------|---------|------|---------|------|---------|------|----------|------------|
| 1973 |      | 4492 |    | 1 |      | 0.22 |       |       |
| 1974 | 1030 | 3494 | 0  | 2 | 0    | 0.57 | 0.59  | -0.59 |
| 1975 | 1030 | 3494 | 1  | 3 | 0.97 | 0.86 | 0.89  | 0.11  |
| 1976 |      | 4492 |    | 3 |      | 0.67 |       |       |
| 1977 | 1224 | 4204 | 0  | 4 | 0    | 0.95 | 1.16  | -1.16 |
| 1978 | 1224 | 4204 | 0  | 2 | 0    | 0.48 | 0.59  | -0.59 |
| 1979 | 1224 | 4204 | 0  | 2 | 0    | 0.48 | 0.59  | -0.59 |
| 1980 | 1224 | 4204 | 0  | 1 | 0    | 0.24 | 0.29  | -0.29 |
| 1981 | 1224 | 4204 | 1  | 2 | 0.82 | 0.48 | 0.59  | 0.41  |
| 1982 | 1224 | 4204 | 1  | 3 | 0.82 | 0.71 | 0.87  | 0.13  |
| 1983 | 1224 | 5048 | 1  | 2 | 0.82 | 0.40 | 0.49  | 0.51  |
| 1984 | 1224 | 5891 | 3  | 2 | 2.45 | 0.34 | 0.42  | 2.58  |
| 1985 | 1224 | 5891 | 0  | 4 | 0    | 0.68 | 0.83  | -0.83 |
| 1986 | 1224 | 5891 | 2  | 2 | 1.63 | 0.34 | 0.42  | 1.58  |
| 1987 | 1224 | 5891 | 0  | 2 | 0    | 0.34 | 0.42  | -0.42 |
| 1988 | 1224 | 5875 | 1  | 3 | 0.82 | 0.51 | 0.62  | 0.38  |
| 1989 | 1227 | 6296 | 0  | 0 | 0    | 0    | 0     | 0     |
| 1990 | 1236 | 6082 | 2  | 2 | 1.62 | 0.33 | 0.41  | 1.59  |
| 1991 | 1240 | 6613 | 1  | 4 | 0.81 | 0.60 | 0.74  | 0.26  |
| 1992 | 1280 | 6479 | 0  | 1 | 0    | 0.15 | 0.19  | -0.19 |
| 1993 | 1375 | 6268 | 2  | 1 | 1.45 | 0.16 | 0.22  | 1.78  |
| 1994 | 1360 | 6138 | 1  | 2 | 0.74 | 0.33 | 0.45  | 0.55  |
| 1995 | 1341 | 4982 | 2  | 1 | 1.49 | 0.20 | 0.27  | 1.73  |
| 1996 | 1329 | 3807 | 2  | 0 | 1.50 | 0    | 0     | 2.00  |
| 1997 | 1329 | 3661 | 4  | 1 | 3.01 | 0.27 | 0.36  | 3.64  |
| 1998 | 1345 | 3499 | 3  | 1 | 2.23 | 0.29 | 0.39  | 2.61  |
| total |     |      | 27 | 51 |     |      | 11.80 | 15.20 |
|       |     |      | observed |  |     |      | expected | difference |

Table 8.23. The excess number of deaths per year among Shipman's patients, males aged 65-74 years. The figures include only MCCDs issued for deaths occurring in the patient's home or on practice premises.

| Year | Number of males 65–74 | | Number of deaths | | Deaths/s 1000 pt | | Expected | Difference |
|------|---------|-----------|---------|-----------|---------|-----------|----------|------------|
|      | Shipman | Comp. GPs | Shipman | Comp. GPs | Shipman | Comp. GPs |          |            |
| 1973 |         | 438       |         | 6         |         | 13.70     |          |            |
| 1974 | 97      | 341       | 0       | 3         | 0       | 8.80      | 0.85     | -0.85      |
| 1975 | 97      | 341       | 1       | 11        | 10.31   | 32.26     | 3.13     | -2.13      |
| 1976 |         | 438       |         | 6         |         | 13.70     |          |            |
| 1977 | 95      | 410       | 0       | 8         | 0       | 19.51     | 1.85     | -1.85      |
| 1978 | 95      | 410       | 5       | 8         | 52.63   | 19.51     | 1.85     | 3.15       |
| 1979 | 95      | 410       | 1       | 11        | 10.53   | 26.83     | 2.55     | -1.55      |
| 1980 | 95      | 410       | 4       | 6         | 42.11   | 14.63     | 1.39     | 2.61       |
| 1981 | 95      | 410       | 1       | 9         | 10.53   | 21.95     | 2.09     | -1.09      |
| 1982 | 95      | 410       | 2       | 9         | 21.05   | 21.95     | 2.09     | -0.09      |
| 1983 | 95      | 492       | 1       | 2         | 10.53   | 4.07      | 0.39     | 0.61       |
| 1984 | 95      | 574       | 2       | 10        | 21.05   | 17.42     | 1.66     | 0.34       |
| 1985 | 95      | 574       | 2       | 4         | 21.05   | 6.97      | 0.66     | 1.34       |
| 1986 | 95      | 574       | 1       | 5         | 10.53   | 8.71      | 0.83     | 0.17       |
| 1987 | 95      | 574       | 1       | 5         | 10.53   | 8.71      | 0.83     | 0.17       |
| 1988 | 95      | 569       | 1       | 7         | 10.53   | 12.30     | 1.17     | -0.17      |
| 1989 | 99      | 627       | 4       | 9         | 40.40   | 14.35     | 1.42     | 2.58       |
| 1990 | 91      | 629       | 0       | 4         | 0       | 6.36      | 0.58     | -0.58      |
| 1991 | 92      | 663       | 1       | 3         | 10.87   | 4.52      | 0.42     | 0.58       |
| 1992 | 97      | 649       | 1       | 5         | 10.31   | 7.70      | 0.75     | 0.25       |
| 1993 | 107     | 655       | 2       | 3         | 18.69   | 4.58      | 0.49     | 1.51       |
| 1994 | 97      | 676       | 0       | 6         | 0       | 8.88      | 0.86     | -0.86      |
| 1995 | 87      | 553       | 3       | 2         | 34.48   | 3.62      | 0.31     | 2.69       |
| 1996 | 89      | 400       | 2       | 2         | 22.47   | 5.00      | 0.45     | 1.55       |
| 1997 | 86      | 384       | 1       | 1         | 11.63   | 2.60      | 0.22     | 0.78       |
| 1998 | 99      | 350       | 0       | 0         | 0       | 0         | 0        | 0          |
| total |        |           | 36 observed | 145  |         |           | 26.84 expected | 9.16 difference |

Table 8.24. The excess number of deaths per year among Shipman's patients, females aged 65–74 years. The figures include only MCCDs issued for deaths occurring in the patient's home or on practice premises.

| Year | Number of females 65–74 | | Number of deaths | | Deaths/s 1000 pt | | Expected | Difference |
|------|---------|-----------|---------|-----------|---------|-----------|----------|-----------|
|      | Shipman | Comp. GPs | Shipman | Comp. GPs | Shipman | Comp. GPs |          |           |
| 1973 |         | 569       |         | 1         |         | 1.76      |          |           |
| 1974 | 127     | 442       | 1       | 5         | 7.87    | 11.31     | 1.44     | -0.44     |
| 1975 | 127     | 442       | 6       | 2         | 47.24   | 4.52      | 0.57     | 5.43      |
| 1976 |         | 569       |         | 6         |         | 10.54     |          |           |
| 1977 | 123     | 532       | 0       | 3         | 0       | 5.64      | 0.69     | -.69      |
| 1978 | 123     | 532       | 3       | 4         | 24.39   | 7.52      | 0.92     | 2.08      |
| 1979 | 123     | 532       | 4       | 4         | 32.52   | 7.52      | 0.92     | 3.08      |
| 1980 | 123     | 532       | 0       | 1         | 0       | 1.88      | 0.23     | -0.23     |
| 1981 | 123     | 532       | 2       | 3         | 16.26   | 5.64      | 0.69     | 1.31      |
| 1982 | 123     | 532       | 2       | 2         | 16.26   | 3.76      | 0.46     | 1.54      |
| 1983 | 123     | 639       | 0       | 7         | 0       | 10.95     | 1.35     | -1.35     |
| 1984 | 123     | 746       | 4       | 6         | 32.52   | 8.04      | 0.99     | 3.01      |
| 1985 | 123     | 746       | 6       | 6         | 48.78   | 8.04      | 0.99     | 5.01      |
| 1986 | 123     | 746       | 1       | 6         | 8.13    | 8.04      | 0.99     | 0.01      |
| 1987 | 123     | 746       | 3       | 3         | 24.39   | 4.02      | 0.49     | 2.51      |
| 1988 | 124     | 738       | 1       | 2         | 8.06    | 2.71      | 0.34     | 0.66      |
| 1989 | 128     | 814       | 1       | 3         | 7.81    | 3.69      | 0.47     | 0.53      |
| 1990 | 118     | 817       | 1       | 2         | 8.47    | 2.45      | 0.29     | 0.71      |
| 1991 | 115     | 868       | 0       | 3         | 0       | 3.46      | 0.40     | -0.40     |
| 1992 | 127     | 859       | 1       | 5         | 7.87    | 5.82      | 0.74     | 0.26      |
| 1993 | 131     | 868       | 4       | 3         | 30.53   | 3.46      | 0.45     | 3.55      |
| 1994 | 134     | 856       | 2       | 3         | 14.93   | 3.50      | 0.47     | 1.53      |
| 1995 | 120     | 711       | 8       | 2         | 66.67   | 2.81      | 0.34     | 7.66      |
| 1996 | 122     | 512       | 3       | 3         | 24.59   | 5.86      | 0.71     | 2.29      |
| 1997 | 120     | 493       | 9       | 1         | 75.00   | 2.03      | 0.24     | 8.76      |
| 1998 | 113     | 463       | 6       | 1         | 53.10   | 2.16      | 0.24     | 5.76      |
| total |        |           | 68 observed | 87 |       |           | 15.42 expected | 52.58 difference |

**Table 8.25. The excess number of deaths per year among Shipman's patients, males aged 75 years or above. The figures include only MCCDs issued for deaths occurring in the patient's home or on practice premises.**

| Year | Number of males 75/+ | | Number of deaths | | Deaths/s 1000 pt | | Expected | Difference |
|------|---------|-----------|---------|-----------|---------|-----------|----------|-----------|
| | Shipman | Comp. GPs | Shipman | Comp. GPs | Shipman | Comp. GPs | | |
| 1973 | | 249 | | 9 | | 36.14 | | |
| 1974 | 57 | 194 | 0 | 5 | 0 | 25.77 | 1.47 | -1.47 |
| 1975 | 57 | 194 | 3 | 12 | 52.63 | 61.86 | 3.53 | -0.53 |
| 1976 | | 249 | | 7 | | 28.11 | | |
| 1977 | 67 | 233 | 1 | 15 | 14.93 | 64.38 | 4.31 | -3.31 |
| 1978 | 67 | 233 | 5 | 12 | 74.63 | 51.50 | 3.45 | 1.55 |
| 1979 | 67 | 233 | 3 | 3 | 44.78 | 12.88 | 0.86 | 2.14 |
| 1980 | 67 | 233 | 3 | 2 | 44.78 | 8.58 | 0.57 | 2.43 |
| 1981 | 67 | 233 | 4 | 4 | 59.70 | 17.17 | 1.15 | 2.85 |
| 1982 | 67 | 233 | 5 | 6 | 74.63 | 25.75 | 1.73 | 3.27 |
| 1983 | 67 | 280 | 3 | 13 | 44.78 | 46.43 | 3.11 | -0.11 |
| 1984 | 67 | 327 | 5 | 8 | 74.63 | 24.46 | 1.64 | 3.36 |
| 1985 | 67 | 327 | 5 | 10 | 74.63 | 30.58 | 2.05 | 2.95 |
| 1986 | 67 | 327 | 2 | 12 | 29.85 | 36.70 | 2.46 | -0.46 |
| 1987 | 67 | 327 | 3 | 16 | 44.78 | 48.93 | 3.28 | -0.28 |
| 1988 | 67 | 319 | 3 | 6 | 44.78 | 18.81 | 1.26 | 1.74 |
| 1989 | 65 | 370 | 3 | 8 | 46.15 | 21.62 | 1.41 | 1.59 |
| 1990 | 64 | 362 | 0 | 5 | 0 | 13.81 | 0.88 | -0.88 |
| 1991 | 64 | 377 | 0 | 4 | 0 | 10.61 | 0.68 | -0.68 |
| 1992 | 63 | 383 | 0 | 5 | 0 | 13.05 | 0.82 | -0.82 |
| 1993 | 60 | 377 | 3 | 3 | 50.00 | 7.96 | 0.48 | 2.52 |
| 1994 | 64 | 369 | 1 | 4 | 15.63 | 10.84 | 0.69 | 0.31 |
| 1995 | 64 | 347 | 8 | 5 | 125.00 | 14.41 | 0.92 | 7.08 |
| 1996 | 64 | 291 | 8 | 3 | 125.00 | 10.31 | 0.66 | 7.34 |
| 1997 | 67 | 277 | 2 | 2 | 29.85 | 7.22 | 0.48 | 1.52 |
| 1998 | 64 | 274 | 2 | 3 | 31.25 | 10.95 | 0.70 | 1.30 |
| total | | | 72 | 182 | | | 38.59 | 33.41 |
| | | | observed | | | | expected | Difference |

| | Table 8.26. The excess number of deaths per year among Shipman's patients, females aged 75 years or above. The figures include only MCCDs issued for deaths occurring in the patient's home or on practice premises. | | | | | | | |

| Year | Number of females 75/+ | | Number of deaths | | Deaths/s 1000 pt | | Expected | Difference |
|------|---------|------|---------|------|---------|------|----------|-----------|
| | Shipman | Comp. GPs | Shipman | Comp. GPs | Shipman | Comp. GPs | | |
| 1973 | | 477 | | 14 | | 29.35 | | |
| 1974 | 104 | 371 | 1 | 10 | 9.62 | 26.95 | 2.80 | -1.80 |
| 1975 | 104 | 371 | 4 | 10 | 38.46 | 26.95 | 2.80 | 1.20 |
| 1976 | | 477 | | 12 | | 25.16 | | |
| 1977 | 121 | 447 | 2 | 5 | 16.53 | 11.19 | 1.35 | 0.65 |
| 1978 | 121 | 447 | 6 | 11 | 49.59 | 24.60 | 2.98 | 3.02 |
| 1979 | 121 | 447 | 10 | 13 | 82.64 | 29.08 | 3.52 | 6.48 |
| 1980 | 121 | 447 | 7 | 14 | 57.85 | 31.32 | 3.79 | 3.21 |
| 1981 | 121 | 447 | 6 | 12 | 49.59 | 26.85 | 3.24 | 2.76 |
| 1982 | 121 | 447 | 3 | 9 | 24.79 | 20.13 | 2.44 | 0.56 |
| 1983 | 121 | 536 | 2 | 11 | 16.53 | 20.52 | 2.48 | -0.48 |
| 1984 | 121 | 626 | 9 | 18 | 74.38 | 28.75 | 3.48 | 5.52 |
| 1985 | 121 | 626 | 7 | 10 | 57.85 | 15.97 | 1.93 | 5.07 |
| 1986 | 121 | 626 | 6 | 10 | 49.59 | 15.97 | 1.93 | 4.07 |
| 1987 | 121 | 626 | 5 | 7 | 41.32 | 11.18 | 1.35 | 3.65 |
| 1988 | 121 | 611 | 10 | 11 | 82.64 | 18.00 | 2.18 | 7.82 |
| 1989 | 117 | 716 | 7 | 7 | 59.83 | 9.78 | 1.14 | 5.86 |
| 1990 | 116 | 694 | 2 | 8 | 17.24 | 11.53 | 1.34 | 0.66 |
| 1991 | 116 | 798 | 4 | 2 | 34.48 | 2.51 | 0.29 | 3.71 |
| 1992 | 110 | 781 | 0 | 6 | 0 | 7.68 | 0.84 | -0.84 |
| 1993 | 102 | 753 | 9 | 4 | 88.24 | 5.31 | 0.54 | 8.46 |
| 1994 | 101 | 730 | 6 | 6 | 59.41 | 8.22 | 0.83 | 5.17 |
| 1995 | 105 | 635 | 11 | 6 | 104.76 | 9.45 | 0.99 | 10.01 |
| 1996 | 94 | 489 | 20 | 3 | 212.77 | 6.13 | 0.58 | 19.42 |
| 1997 | 87 | 505 | 22 | 2 | 252.87 | 3.96 | 0.34 | 21.66 |
| 1998 | 77 | 514 | 10 | 2 | 129.87 | 3.89 | 0.30 | 9.70 |
| total | | | 169 observed | 223 | | | 43.46 expected | 125.54 difference |

Tables 8.15-26 highlight the total number of excess deaths and the patient groups that account for most of them. The total number of MCCDs issued by Shipman irrespective of place of death was 521, but the expected number was 223.4, a difference of 297.6 (95% confidence interval 254 to 345 (Gardner and Altman, 1989). The number of MCCDs issued by Shipman for deaths occurring at home was 397, but the expected number was 160.8, a difference of 236.2 (95% confidence interval 198 to 277). Although it cannot be assumed that no deaths among people in residential or nursing homes should be viewed with concern, the proportion of such deaths classified as suspicious was low. Therefore, the excess numbers of deaths occurring at home or on practice premises is more likely to reflect the true number that should give rise to concern.

The patient group accounting for most excess deaths was females aged 75 or over, followed by females aged 65-74. Males aged 75 or above accounted for the third highest number of excess deaths, followed by females under aged 65. The excess numbers of deaths were highest from 1995, but an excess among females aged 75 or above was evident from 1977 onwards. The figures for 1974 and 1975 should be treated with caution since they relate to incomplete years worked. Nevertheless, in 1975 there was an excess of deaths among females aged 65–74.

The figures do not indicate a sustained period when the numbers of deaths were at the expected level. In order to identify the point at which the numbers of excess deaths distinctly diverged from the expected level, graphs were plotted of the cumulative numbers of excess deaths. The findings are shown in Figures 8.7–8.9. They relate to deaths at home or on practice premises only, and indicate for each year the accumulated number of excess deaths. In each graph, the axis placed at zero for the number of excess deaths is the level that would have been expected if death rates among Shipman's patients had been the same as among patients of the comparison practitioners.

Figure 8.7 presents the findings for males and females aged under 65 years. For males, there is no accumulation of excess deaths. However, among females, the numbers accumulate from 1986 onwards.

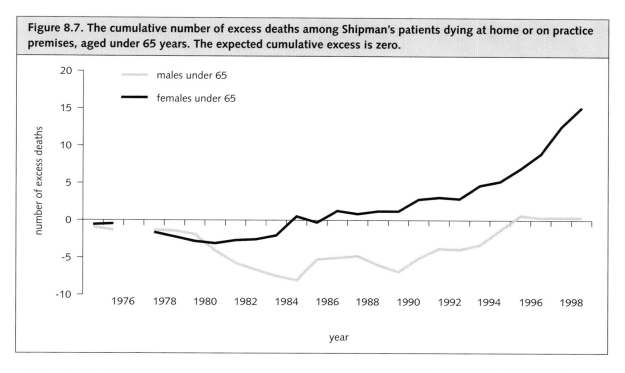

**Figure 8.7. The cumulative number of excess deaths among Shipman's patients dying at home or on practice premises, aged under 65 years. The expected cumulative excess is zero.**

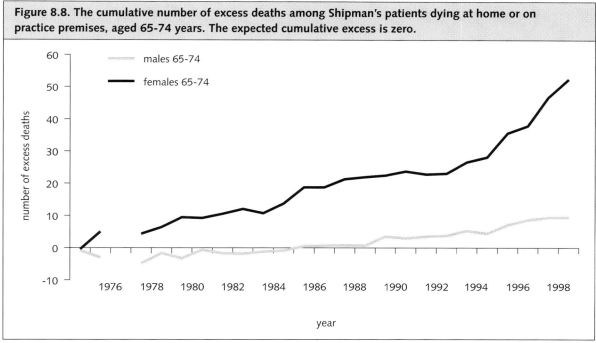

**Figure 8.8. The cumulative number of excess deaths among Shipman's patients dying at home or on practice premises, aged 65-74 years. The expected cumulative excess is zero.**

The pattern for patients aged 65–74 shows an accumulation of excess deaths among males from 1989, and among females from 1975 (Figure 8.8). In those aged 75 or above, the excess accumulated from 1978 among females, and from 1981 among males (Figure 8.9).

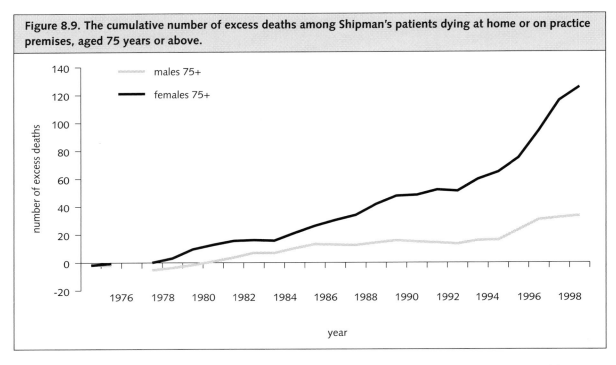

**Figure 8.9. The cumulative number of excess deaths among Shipman's patients dying at home or on practice premises, aged 75 years or above.**

The findings therefore indicate that the large excess of deaths from 1995 onwards was not a sudden new feature of Shipman's clinical practice, but an exacerbation of a trend that can be traced to his earliest years as a general practitioner.

## 8.3.7. Certified cause of death

Shipman was more likely to give heart conditions, stroke and old age as the cause of death than the comparison practitioners (Table 8.27).

**Table 8.27. The numbers of deaths certified as caused by different groups of conditions by Shipman and the comparison practitioners. ($X_4^2 = 127.7$; $p - 0.000$).**

|  | Shipman (%) | | Comparison practitioners | |
|---|---|---|---|---|
|  | N | % | N | % |
| heart conditions | 177 | (34.0) | 319 | (28.1) |
| stroke | 93 | (17.9) | 130 | (11.4) |
| cancer | 91 | (17.5) | 337 | (29.7) |
| old age | 88 | (16.9) | 50 | (4.4) |
| other | 72 | (13.8) | 300 | (26.4) |

However, the differences varied during Shipman's working life. He was more likely to indicate heart conditions or stroke as the cause of death in the years after 1987 (Figure 8.10). In earlier years, his use of old age or similar terms as the cause of death was much greater than the comparison practitioners (Figure 8.11).

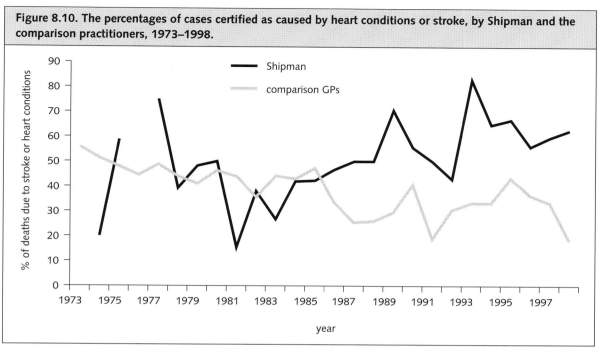

**Figure 8.10. The percentages of cases certified as caused by heart conditions or stroke, by Shipman and the comparison practitioners, 1973–1998.**

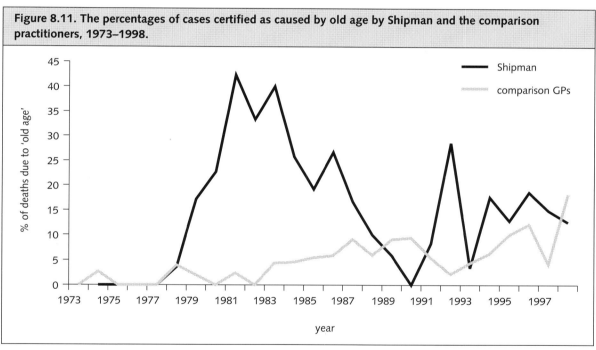

**Figure 8.11. The percentages of cases certified as caused by old age by Shipman and the comparison practitioners, 1973–1998.**

## 8.3.6. Cremation

A marginally greater proportion of deaths certified by Shipman was followed by cremations, 392 (75.2%) of Shipman's patients and 802 (70.6%) of the comparison practitioners' being cremated. There was no clear trend from year to year (Figure 8.12).

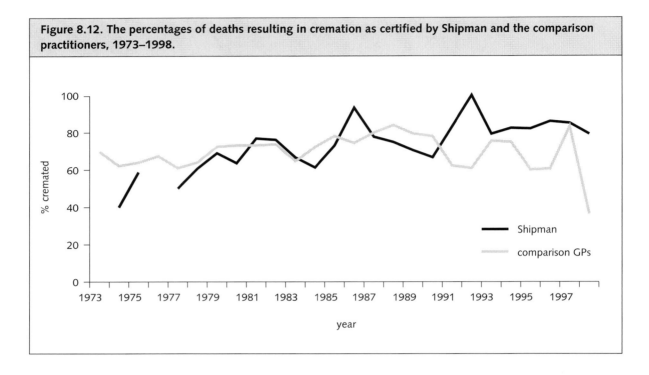

**Figure 8.12. The percentages of deaths resulting in cremation as certified by Shipman and the comparison practitioners, 1973–1998.**

## 8.3.7. Day of the week

The number of deaths certified by general practitioners as occurring on different days of the week can be expected to be similar. Although some general practitioners may delegate out of hours care on certain days of the week (for example, weekends), the MCCDs for any deaths that could be certified would still be completed by the patient's general practitioner on the next working day. On the other hand, the daily schedule of a general practitioner will influence the amount of time available on any particular day for routine home visits. For example, there would be less time for such visits on days in which the practitioner offers additional clinics or consulting sessions. It is possible, therefore, that on certain week days, Shipman would have had more time to initiate visits to patients in their homes.

Table 8.28 presents information about the numbers of deaths on each day of the week certified by Shipman and the comparison practitioners. Shipman certified a higher proportion of deaths on Mondays, Tuesdays and Fridays, with the lowest proportion occurring on Saturdays and Sundays. The comparison practitioners had a more consistent distribution. It is difficult to identify a reasonable clinical or administrative explanation for Shipman's pattern.

Table 8.28. The numbers (%) of deaths on different days of the week certified by Shipman and the comparison practitioners, 1973–1998. ($X_6^2 = 16.0$; $p - 0.014$).

| Week day | Shipman | | Comparison GPs | |
|---|---|---|---|---|
| | N | % | N | % |
| Monday | 87 | 16.7 | 152 | 13.4 |
| Tuesday | 95 | 18.2 | 167 | 14.7 |
| Wednesday | 70 | 13.4 | 184 | 16.2 |
| Thursday | 80 | 15.4 | 178 | 15.7 |
| Friday | 84 | 16.1 | 150 | 13.2 |
| Saturday | 59 | 11.3 | 167 | 14.7 |
| Sunday | 46 | 8.8 | 138 | 12.1 |
| Totals | 521 | 100 | 1136 | 100 |

## 8.3.8. Month

In contrast, there was no difference between Shipman and the comparison practitioners in the numbers of deaths for which they issued MCCDs in each month. A greater proportion of deaths occurred during the winter months (December – March, see Table 8.29). The Table only includes data relating to full years worked by Shipman (1978–1997).

Table 8.29. The numbers (%) of MCCDs issued by Shipman and the comparison practitioners each month, 1978–1997. ($X_{11}^2 = 12.1$; $p - 0.036$).

| | Shipman (%) | | Comparison practitioners | |
|---|---|---|---|---|
| | N | % | N | % |
| January | 46 | 9.8 | 104 | 11.5 |
| February | 43 | 9.1 | 75 | 8.3 |
| March | 48 | 10.2 | 79 | 8.7 |
| April | 42 | 8.9 | 67 | 7.4 |
| May | 46 | 9.8 | 70 | 7.7 |
| June | 31 | 6.6 | 68 | 7.5 |
| July | 36 | 7.6 | 69 | 7.6 |
| August | 30 | 6.4 | 59 | 6.5 |
| September | 35 | 7.4 | 69 | 7.6 |
| October | 29 | 6.2 | 81 | 8.9 |
| November | 39 | 8.3 | 70 | 7.7 |
| December | 46 | 9.8 | 97 | 10.7 |
| Totals | 471 | 100 | 908 | 100 |

## 8.3.9. Variation in the numbers of deaths

In some years, Shipman issued relatively few MCCDs – 1974, 1977, 1983, 1986, 1990, 1991 and 1992. In both 1974 and 1977 he worked for only part of the year, and therefore only a small number of MCCDs would be anticipated, but in the other years he worked throughout all twelve months.

In 1983, he issued 15 MCCDs, a number that would not have been unexpected when compared to the numbers issued by the comparison practitioners (Table 8.1). A relatively high proportion were in the age group 75-84 (Table 8.3) and were certified as due to old age or similar causes (Figure 8.11). Ten (66.7%) were females. These are features established as typical of the convictions, but it should also be noted that only eight (53.3%) died at home (Figure 8.2) and of the five cremation forms still available for review, four led to classification as not suspicious and one as moderately suspicious. Therefore, the number of deaths in 1983 that should give cause for concern is likely to be lower than in other years.

In 1986, Shipman issued 16 MCCDs. A high proportion were in the 75-84 age group, 11 (73.3%) were females, and seven (46.7%) were certified as due to heart conditions. Thirteen (86.7%) died at home, and on review of the surviving cremation forms and clinical records, eight deaths (57.1%) were classified as highly suspicious and two (14.3%) as moderately suspicious (Table 8.30). Thus, although the total numbers of deaths in 1986 may not have been particularly high, the presence of the typical features is cause for concern.

There was a marked decline in the annual number of deaths between 1990 and 1992, and the numbers classified as suspicious in these years were also low (Table 8.30). The numbers in the 75 to 84 age group were three (33.3%) in 1990, seven (58.3%) in 1991, and two (28.6%) in 1992. The numbers of females in each year were seven (77.8%), eight (66.7%) and five (71.4%) respectively. The numbers certified as due to stroke or heart conditions were five (55.6%), six (50%) and three (42%) respectively. Thus, although it cannot be assumed that no death in these years should give cause for concern, the number of such deaths was low. It is notable that this decline in numbers of deaths and numbers classified as suspicious took place in the two years leading up to, and the year after, Shipman's departure from the group practice to set up in practice alone.

## 8.3.10. Cases classified according to level of suspicion

The annual numbers of cases that were classified according to the level of suspicion as determined from review of the clinical records and/or cremation forms are shown in Table 8.30. The figures include the 15 convictions. The variation in the numbers classified as moderately or highly suspicious substantially accounts for the annual variation in the total numbers of MCCDs issued. A total of 166 (57.6%) of the 288 deaths between 1985 and 1998 with either records and/or cremation forms still available were classified as highly suspicious.

**Table 8.30. The annual numbers of cases classified according to level of suspicion about the circumstances of death, 1985–1998. (n=288).**

| Year | None | | Moderate | | High | | Total n | All MCCDs issued by Shipman |
|---|---|---|---|---|---|---|---|---|
| | n | % | n | % | n | % | | |
| 1985 | 9 | 47.4 | 3 | 15.8 | 7 | 36.8 | 19 | 26 |
| 1986 | 4 | 28.6 | 2 | 14.3 | 8 | 57.1 | 14 | 16 |
| 1987 | 6 | 42.9 | 1 | 7.1 | 7 | 50.0 | 14 | 18 |
| 1988 | 6 | 40.0 | 2 | 13.3 | 7 | 46.7 | 15 | 20 |
| 1989 | 2 | 16.7 | 1 | 8.3 | 9 | 75.0 | 12 | 17 |
| 1990 | 6 | 85.7 | 0 | | 1 | 14.3 | 7 | 9 |
| 1991 | 6 | 54.5 | 3 | 27.3 | 2 | 18.2 | 11 | 12 |
| 1992 | 3 | 42.9 | 2 | 28.6 | 2 | 28.6 | 7 | 7 |
| 1993 | 8 | 30.8 | 4 | 15.4 | 14 | 53.8 | 26 | 29 |
| 1994 | 5 | 33.3 | 1 | 6.7 | 9 | 60.0 | 15 | 17 |
| 1995 | 5 | 13.5 | 10 | 27.0 | 22 | 59.5 | 37 | 39 |
| 1996 | 8 | 19.5 | 6 | 14.6 | 27 | 65.9 | 41 | 43 |
| 1997 | 7 | 15.2 | 4 | 8.7 | 35 | 76.1 | 46 | 47 |
| 1998 | 4 | 16.7 | 4 | 16.7 | 16 | 66.7 | 24 | 24 |
| Total | 79 | 27.4 | 43 | 14.9 | 166 | 57.6 | 288 | 324 |

Clinical records or cremation forms were not available for 36 cases, and therefore these cases could not be classified according to the degree of suspicion about the circumstances of death. However, had records or cremation forms been available, it is likely that a proportion of these would have been classified as suspicious. If the annual percentages in the none, moderately or highly suspicious groups among cases with records or cremation forms are assumed to apply to the cases without this information in each year, it can be estimated that an additional 18 cases would have been classified as highly suspicious.

Thus, on this basis 184 of the 324 cases from 1985 would have been classified as highly suspicious. The number of excess deaths among patients dying at home 1985-1998 was 199 (Tables 8.21-8.26). This finding suggests that the most likely number of excess deaths about which there should be concern is that indicated by the excess among patients dying at home.

A further notable aspect of the annual numbers of deaths is the steep increase from 1995 onwards (Table 8.1). Documentary evidence obtained from clinical records and/or cremation forms was available for most cases in these years, and the proportion classified as either moderately or highly suspicious was above 80% in each year. One hundred deaths in this period (1995-1998) were classified as highly suspicious, and 24 as moderately suspicious.

## 8.3.11. Deaths in 1998

Shipman was arrested and therefore ceased clinical practice on 7th September 1998. He issued 24 MCCDs in 1998, the last one being issued in June, and most being issued in the early months of the year. Thus, 18 were issued between January and the end of March, 13 of which were classified as highly suspicious. The first investigation into Shipman's activities was initiated at the end of March and one possible explanation for the reduction in the numbers of deaths from then onwards is that he might have become aware that concerns had been raised. An attempt to avoid detection may also explain the decline in deaths in 1990 when working in the group practice. However, the available evidence does not contain any indication of what might have triggered such a strategy. One death did occur on practice premises in 1989, but this occurred in March and was followed by several further deaths that were classified as moderately or highly suspicious.

## 8.3.12. Todmorden

Twenty-two of the 521 MCCDs issued by Shipman in his career as a general practitioner were completed for patients who died in Todmorden. A local investigation has raised concerns about the possibility that Shipman murdered some patients in the 19 months he spent in the practice in Todmorden (see Section 2.4). The information available to the audit about the deaths in 1974 and 1975 was limited to that contained in death notifications, and therefore any conclusions must be tentative.

The precise date that Shipman ceased to work in Todmorden is uncertain, but is believed to have been some time in September 1975. Thus, the 17 deaths that occurred in 1975 took place over a nine month period, and the equivalent annual death rate would have been 23. This is a higher figure than that of any of the other comparison doctors in Todmorden (Table 2.2).

Shipman issued only five MCCDs in 1974, two of which related to deaths in a local hospital. However, in 1975 the patterns of deaths are suggestive of some of the features found typical at the trial. Tests of statistical significance are not reported since the number of cases is too small.

Of the 17 patients, 16 (94.1%) died at home. The comparison practitioners issued MCCDs for 50 patients during 1975, and 43 (86.0%) of these died at home. Eleven (64.7%) of Shipman's patients were female, but only 18 (36.0%) of the comparison practitioners' patients were female. The age groups were also different (Table 8.31). In 1975, nine (52.9%) deaths were certified by Shipman as due to heart conditions, but the equivalent number for the comparison practitioners was 18 (36%). The comparison practitioners were more likely to give stroke or other conditions as the cause of death.

| Table 8.31 Numbers (%) of patients of Shipman and comparison practitioners, in different age groups, 1975. | | | | |
|---|---|---|---|---|
| Age group (yrs) | Shipman | | Comparison GPs | |
| 0–50 | 0 | | 3 | 6.0 |
| 51–64 | 2 | 11.8 | 8 | 16.0 |
| 65–74 | 8 | 47.1 | 14 | 28.0 |
| 75–84 | 3 | 17.6 | 18 | 36.0 |
| 85 or above | 4 | 23.5 | 7 | 14.0 |
| | 17 | | 50 | |

Three deaths certified by Shipman in January 1975 occurred on the same day, and two deaths occurred on the same day in March. There was a difference between Shipman and the comparison practitioners in the numbers of deaths on different days of the week, with a greater proportion of Shipman's deaths occurring on Mondays and Tuesdays. However, in view of the small numbers of cases involved, it would be unwise to place weight on this finding.

In addition to this limited information about the presence of the typical features, four other factors should be taken into account in considering whether there are reasons to be concerned about deaths in Todmorden in 1974 and 1975. First, the numbers of deaths in Hyde were higher than expected from 1978, the earliest full year in which Shipman practised in the town. The age groups and proportion of females among the excess numbers of deaths from 1978 were such as to give cause for concern (see Figures 8.7-8.9). Thus, it has not been possible to identify a period in Hyde before which there can be no cause for concern about Shipman's activities.

Second, the investigation by *Todmorden News and Advertiser* included a report from a past patient of Shipman that raised the possibility that he may have intended to murder her.

Third, a report prepared by a forensic psychologist at the request of Greater Manchester Police in January 1998 concluded that Shipman's drive to murder 'would be likely to have been there from at least adolescence onwards, would have found expression long before the accused's current age (dependent on opportunity), and would be likely to escalate in frequency over time'.

Fourth, it was established that Shipman had illegally obtained supplies of pethidine injections. He admitted taking this medication himself, but it cannot be ruled out that he administered some of this medication to patients.

There are, therefore, reasons for concern about the cause of some deaths in Todmorden. However, such concern rests on the very limited evidence obtained from death notifications and inferences from other observations, and can only be tentative. Evidence from other sources would be required to substantiate or refute the concerns.

# 8.4 Conclusions

The analyses of data obtained from the MCCDs issued by Shipman during his career as a general practitioner have revealed distinctive findings:

- Among Shipman's patients, there was an excess in relation to the patients of the comparison practitioners of 297 deaths (95% confidence interval 254-345).

- Among patients who died at home or on practice premises, the excess number of deaths was 236 (95% confidence interval 198-277).

- The excess was highest among females aged 75 and above, second highest among females aged 65–74, and third highest among males aged 75 and above.

- Higher proportions of Shipman's patients died between the ages of 75 and 84, were female, died at home or in the practice and were certified as dying from heart conditions, stroke or old age than the patients of the comparison practitioners.

Thus, in addition to their excess numbers, deaths among Shipman's patients exhibited some of the features typical of the convictions – age and sex, place of death and certified causes of death. Furthermore, in the years when clinical records or cremation forms were available, the numbers of cases classified as highly or moderately suspicious were relatively similar to the estimated excess of deaths occuring at home.

There were variations in the annual numbers of deaths. They were low leading up to and after Shipman's move to the single-handed practice (1990-92), but increased steeply from 1993-1998. The numbers were also relatively high from 1978 to 1982, and from 1984 to 1989, although the levels in these years were lower than 1993 onwards.

It was not possible to identify a sustained period before which Shipman's death rates were similar to other local practitioners. Therefore, although the available evidence is limited, there must be concern about the circumstances leading to some of the deaths whilst Shipman worked in Todmorden.

# Nine: Prospective analysis of deaths of patients registered with Shipman from 1987

## 9.1  Background

The numbers of deaths shown in Tables 2.1 and 2.2 relate to MCCDs that were issued by general practitioners, and exclude deaths in hospital or outside the district. It is possible, therefore, that an observed excess in the numbers of MCCDs issued might be explained by the proportions of patients dying in hospital or elsewhere under the care of other doctors. For example, if Shipman was more likely to care for patients in their own homes rather than admit them to hospital, the total numbers of deaths among his patients would be similar to other practitioners, but the proportion dying in hospital would be lower. Patient preference may also be a factor in decisions about hospital admission, and in some cases Shipman did indicate in the clinical records that patients had been reluctant to be admitted to hospital.

The yardstick against which to compare the numbers of MCCDs issued by Shipman in Tables 2.1 and 2.2, and in Section Eight, was the MCCDs issued by a group of local general practitioners. Although the socio-economic characteristics of Shipman's and the comparison practitioners' patients were similar, it is possible, although unlikely, that for some unidentified reason the death rate among the patients of the comparison practitioners was unusually low. If this had been the case, although the numbers of deaths among Shipman's patients may have been normal, the comparison would have suggested an excess. Therefore, a comparison between death rates among Shipman's patients and other groups is required.

In order to address such issues, an investigation of the numbers of deaths among patients registered with Shipman was undertaken.

## 9.2  Method

The information for this component of the audit was provided by the Office for National Statistics (ONS), under the supervision of Peter Goldblatt, Chief Medical Statistician. The first step involved the identification of patients who had been registered with Shipman. Information about patient registration was obtained from West Pennine Health Authority. The details were held on the Exeter system family health services register, and it was possible to track transactions on the register from 1987. Such transactions include the registration of a patient with a general practitioner, and removal from the register as a consequence of registration with another general practitioner, death or other reasons. Thus, the patients included in this aspect of the audit were all those who were registered with Shipman at the beginning of 1987, or who joined Shipman's list subsequently. Care was taken to identify all patients who had been registered with Shipman.

Information about identified patients was submitted to ONS and a search was then made of death registers to identify deaths that had occurred whilst the patient was registered with Shipman. These searches were principally conducted through the National Health Service Central Register (NHSCR). The NHSCR was used to check whether the person was alive, and if deceased to provide the details needed to trace the death records. In calculating the death rate among Shipman's patients, information was used about the numbers of patients registered with him, and the period during which they were registered to produce an estimate of the numbers of person years at risk of death.

In estimating the numbers of deaths that would have been expected, three comparison groups were used. These were the population of England and Wales, deaths among the population of manufacturing districts, and deaths among the population of Tameside. Manufacturing districts are districts in Great Britain classified in the ONS classification of local and health authorities into sets of authorities that share broad population socio-economic characteristics (Bailey et al, 2000). The manufacturing district mortality data were derived from the mean number of deaths between 1991 and 1997. For England and Wales and Tameside, the annual number of deaths of usual residents was related to the respective annual population estimates. The three comparison groups were then used to calculate the number of deaths that would have been expected among Shipman's patients if the rate of death of his patients had been the same as England and Wales, manufacturing districts or Tameside. The calculation took account of the numbers and ages of Shipman's male and female patients, and the period during which they were registered with him in each year.

# 9.3 Findings

Tables 9.1–12 summarise the findings. There was an excess number of deaths among females (all age groups combined) from 1995 to 1998. The lower 95% confidence limit for the annual number of deaths among Shipman's patients was higher than the expected number of deaths as estimated by rates for England and Wales, manufacturing districts and Tameside in these years and also in 1988 and 1993 (Table 9.1). However, in 1987, between 1989 and 1992, and in 1994, the expected numbers of deaths were within the confidence limits of Shipman's numbers of deaths.

Among females aged 65–74, the lower 95% confidence limit of the observed deaths exceeded the expected deaths in 1995, 1997 and 1998 (Table 9.4). Among females aged 75–84, the observed exceeded those expected in 1987, 1993, and 1996–1998 (Table 9.5). Among females aged 85 and over, the observed exceeded the expected in 1988 and 1995–1997 (Table 9.6). There were no differences in the other age groups.

No differences in death rates were identified among males, all age groups combined (Table 9.7). Furthermore, there were no differences in any age group. In comparison with Tameside, there were 98 more deaths than expected among Shipman's female patients and 12 less than expected among males. In comparison with death rates in manufacturing districts, there were 114 deaths more than expected among females and four more deaths than expected among males. In comparison with England and Wales, there were 126 more deaths than expected among females and 21 deaths more than expected among males.

Table 9.1. Observed deaths among Shipman's female patients in all age groups, 1987–1998, showing upper and lower 95% confidence limits. Table includes expected numbers of deaths based on estimates relating to England and Wales, manufacturing districts, and Tameside. SMR = standardised mortality rate among Shipman's patients; CL = confidence limit; Exp = expected.

| Females | All ages Observed deaths | Lower CL | Upper CL | E&W standard Exp | SMR | Manufacturing standard Exp | SMR | Tameside standard Exp | SMR |
|---|---|---|---|---|---|---|---|---|---|
| All years | 341 | 305.8 | 379.2 | 215.1 | 159 | 227.3 | 150 | 243.1 | 140 |
| 1987 | 25 | 16.1 | 36.9 | 17.4 | 144 | 17.4 | 143 | 18.7 | 133 |
| 1988 | 33 | 22.7 | 46.4 | 19.5 | 169 | 19.6 | 168 | 22.2 | 148 |
| 1989 | 18 | 10.6 | 28.5 | 19.5 | 92 | 19.5 | 92 | 22.1 | 81 |
| 1990 | 17 | 9.9 | 27.2 | 19.3 | 88 | 20.2 | 84 | 21.9 | 78 |
| 1991 | 14 | 7.6 | 23.5 | 20.0 | 70 | 20.8 | 67 | 22.0 | 64 |
| 1992 | 13 | 6.9 | 22.3 | 19.9 | 65 | 21.4 | 61 | 21.4 | 61 |
| 1993 | 34 | 23.5 | 47.5 | 20.0 | 170 | 20.8 | 163 | 22.4 | 152 |
| 1994 | 19 | 11.4 | 29.7 | 19.2 | 99 | 21.0 | 90 | 22.6 | 84 |
| 1995 | 43 | 31.1 | 57.9 | 19.3 | 223 | 20.7 | 207 | 22.1 | 194 |
| 1996 | 43 | 31.1 | 57.9 | 17.2 | 250 | 18.9 | 228 | 20.0 | 215 |
| 1997 | 52 | 38.8 | 68.2 | 14.7 | 353 | 16.5 | 316 | 16.5 | 316 |
| 1998 | 30 | 20.2 | 42.8 | 9.2 | 324 | 10.5 | 286 | 11.2 | 267 |

Table 9.2. Observed deaths among Shipman's female patients aged under 45 years, 1987–1998, showing upper and lower 95% confidence limits. Table includes expected numbers of deaths based on estimates relating to England and Wales, manufacturing districts, and Tameside. SMR = standardised mortality rate among Shipman's patients; CL = confidence limit; Exp = expected.

| Females | Under 45 Observed deaths | Lower CL | Upper CL | E&W standard Exp | SMR | Manufacturing standard Exp | SMR | Tameside standard Exp | SMR |
|---|---|---|---|---|---|---|---|---|---|
| All years | 5 | 1.5 | 11.7 | 10.2 | 49 | 11.0 | 45 | 10.6 | 47 |
| 1987 | 0 | 0.0 | 3.7 | 0.9 | 0 | 0.8 | 0 | 0.8 | 0 |
| 1988 | 0 | 0.0 | 3.7 | 1.0 | 0 | 1.0 | 0 | 1.1 | 0 |
| 1989 | 0 | 0.0 | 3.7 | 1.0 | 0 | 1.0 | 0 | 1.1 | 0 |
| 1990 | 0 | 0.0 | 3.7 | 0.9 | 0 | 0.9 | 0 | 1.0 | 0 |
| 1991 | 0 | 0.0 | 3.7 | 0.9 | 0 | 1.0 | 0 | 0.9 | 0 |
| 1992 | 0 | 0.0 | 3.7 | 0.9 | 0 | 1.0 | 0 | 0.9 | 0 |
| 1993 | 1 | 0.0 | 5.6 | 0.9 | 114 | 1.0 | 101 | 0.9 | 107 |
| 1994 | 0 | 0.0 | 3.7 | 0.8 | 0 | 0.9 | 0 | 0.8 | 0 |
| 1995 | 3 | 0.6 | 8.8 | 0.8 | 378 | 0.9 | 332 | 1.0 | 296 |
| 1996 | 0 | 0.0 | 3.7 | 0.8 | 0 | 0.9 | 0 | 0.8 | 0 |
| 1997 | 1 | 0.0 | 5.6 | 0.8 | 124 | 0.9 | 107 | 0.7 | 143 |
| 1998 | 0 | 0.0 | 3.7 | 0.6 | 0 | 0.7 | 0 | 0.6 | 0 |

Table 9.3. Observed deaths among Shipman's female patients aged 45–64, 1987–1998, showing upper and lower 95% confidence limits. Table includes expected numbers of deaths based on estimates relating to England and Wales, manufacturing districts, and Tameside. SMR = standardised mortality rate among Shipman's patients; CL = confidence limit; Exp = expected.

| Females 45–64 | Observed deaths | Lower CL | Upper CL | E&W standard | | Manufacturing standard | | Tameside standard | |
|---|---|---|---|---|---|---|---|---|---|
| | | | | Exp | SMR | Exp | SMR | Exp | SMR |
| All years | 37 | 26.0 | 51.0 | 25.0 | 148 | 27.4 | 135 | 30.7 | 120 |
| 1987 | 2 | 0.2 | 7.3 | 2.0 | 99 | 1.9 | 104 | 2.4 | 82 |
| 1988 | 3 | 0.6 | 8.8 | 2.3 | 131 | 2.2 | 133 | 2.8 | 109 |
| 1989 | 1 | 0.0 | 3.7 | 2.1 | 47 | 2.1 | 47 | 2.9 | 35 |
| 1990 | 3 | 0.6 | 8.8 | 2.1 | 140 | 2.2 | 136 | 2.9 | 102 |
| 1991 | 1 | 0.0 | 3.7 | 2.1 | 47 | 2.3 | 44 | 2.6 | 39 |
| 1992 | 1 | 0.0 | 3.7 | 2.1 | 47 | 2.3 | 43 | 2.4 | 41 |
| 1993 | 3 | 0.6 | 8.8 | 2.2 | 137 | 2.4 | 125 | 2.4 | 123 |
| 1994 | 3 | 0.6 | 8.8 | 2.1 | 140 | 2.5 | 121 | 2.6 | 116 |
| 1995 | 4 | 1.1 | 10.3 | 2.2 | 185 | 2.5 | 160 | 2.7 | 148 |
| 1996 | 6 | 2.1 | 13.1 | 2.1 | 285 | 2.5 | 239 | 2.7 | 223 |
| 1997 | 6 | 2.1 | 13.1 | 2.1 | 289 | 2.5 | 238 | 2.6 | 229 |
| 1998 | 4 | 1.1 | 10.3 | 1.5 | 269 | 1.8 | 218 | 1.7 | 237 |

Table 9.4. Observed deaths among Shipman's female patients aged 65–74, 1987–1998, showing upper and lower 95% confidence limits. Table includes expected numbers of deaths based on estimates relating to England and Wales, manufacturing districts, and Tameside. SMR = standardised mortality rate among Shipman's patients; CL = confidence limit; Exp = expected.

| Females 65–74 | Observed deaths | Lower CL | Upper CL | E&W standard | | Manufacturing standard | | Tameside standard | |
|---|---|---|---|---|---|---|---|---|---|
| | | | | Exp | SMR | Exp | SMR | Exp | SMR |
| All years | 75 | 59.0 | 94.0 | 40.2 | 187 | 45.0 | 167 | 50.3 | 149 |
| 1987 | 5 | 1.6 | 11.7 | 2.9 | 170 | 3.1 | 159 | 3.3 | 151 |
| 1988 | 4 | 1.1 | 10.3 | 3.6 | 112 | 3.8 | 106 | 4.3 | 94 |
| 1989 | 2 | 0.2 | 7.3 | 3.8 | 52 | 4.0 | 49 | 4.4 | 45 |
| 1990 | 7 | 2.8 | 14.5 | 3.7 | 191 | 4.0 | 174 | 4.7 | 149 |
| 1991 | 3 | 0.6 | 8.8 | 3.5 | 85 | 3.9 | 77 | 4.3 | 70 |
| 1992 | 4 | 1.1 | 10.3 | 3.6 | 112 | 4.0 | 99 | 4.5 | 89 |
| 1993 | 5 | 1.6 | 11.7 | 3.8 | 133 | 4.2 | 120 | 4.9 | 102 |
| 1994 | 4 | 1.1 | 10.3 | 3.7 | 108 | 4.3 | 93 | 5.2 | 77 |
| 1995 | 13 | 6.9 | 22.3 | 3.5 | 376 | 3.9 | 330 | 4.4 | 292 |
| 1996 | 5 | 1.6 | 11.7 | 3.2 | 154 | 3.8 | 131 | 4.0 | 126 |
| 1997 | 12 | 6.2 | 21.0 | 3.0 | 401 | 3.6 | 333 | 3.8 | 316 |
| 1998 | 11 | 5.5 | 19.7 | 1.9 | 581 | 2.3 | 474 | 2.5 | 437 |

Table 9.5. Observed deaths among Shipman's female patients aged 75–84, 1987–1998, showing upper and lower 95% confidence limits. Table includes expected numbers of deaths based on estimates relating to England and Wales, manufacturing districts, and Tameside. SMR = standardised mortality rate among Shipman's patients; CL = confidence limit; Exp = expected.

| Females 75–84 | Observed deaths | Lower CL | Upper CL | E&W standard | | Manufacturing standard | | Tameside standard | |
|---|---|---|---|---|---|---|---|---|---|
| | | | | Exp | SMR | Exp | SMR | Exp | SMR |
| All years | 135 | 113.2 | 159.8 | 67.2 | 201 | 70.9 | 190 | 76.1 | 177 |
| 1987 | 14 | 7.6 | 23.5 | 6.4 | 220 | 6.4 | 217 | 6.7 | 210 |
| 1988 | 12 | 6.1 | 21.0 | 6.5 | 184 | 6.7 | 180 | 7.2 | 168 |
| 1989 | 12 | 6.1 | 21.0 | 6.7 | 178 | 6.8 | 176 | 8.1 | 147 |
| 1990 | 4 | 1.1 | 10.3 | 6.8 | 59 | 7.2 | 56 | 7.9 | 51 |
| 1991 | 8 | 3.5 | 15.8 | 7.0 | 114 | 7.3 | 109 | 7.7 | 104 |
| 1992 | 6 | 2.2 | 13.1 | 6.6 | 91 | 7.0 | 85 | 7.0 | 85 |
| 1993 | 15 | 8.3 | 24.8 | 5.8 | 259 | 6.0 | 251 | 6.4 | 235 |
| 1994 | 6 | 2.2 | 13.1 | 5.2 | 116 | 5.6 | 107 | 5.9 | 102 |
| 1995 | 8 | 3.5 | 15.8 | 5.1 | 157 | 5.5 | 145 | 5.8 | 137 |
| 1996 | 18 | 10.6 | 28.5 | 4.7 | 385 | 5.1 | 350 | 5.9 | 303 |
| 1997 | 22 | 13.7 | 33.3 | 4.0 | 550 | 4.5 | 492 | 4.5 | 490 |
| 1998 | 10 | 4.8 | 18.4 | 2.4 | 413 | 2.7 | 367 | 3.0 | 332 |

Table 9.6. Observed deaths among Shipman's female patients aged 85 and over, 1987–1998, showing upper and lower 95% confidence limits. Table includes expected numbers of deaths based on estimates relating to England and Wales, manufacturing districts, and Tameside. SMR = standardised mortality rate among Shipman's patients; CL = confidence limit; Exp = expected.

| Females 85 and over | Observed deaths | Lower CL | Upper CL | E&W standard | | Manufacturing standard | | Tameside standard | |
|---|---|---|---|---|---|---|---|---|---|
| | | | | Exp | SMR | Exp | SMR | Exp | SMR |
| All years | 89 | 71.5 | 109.5 | 72.6 | 123 | 72.9 | 122 | 75.3 | 118 |
| 1987 | 4 | 1.1 | 10.3 | 5.2 | 77 | 5.1 | 78 | 5.5 | 73 |
| 1988 | 14 | 7.6 | 23.5 | 6.1 | 229 | 5.9 | 238 | 6.9 | 201 |
| 1989 | 3 | 0.6 | 8.8 | 5.8 | 52 | 5.6 | 54 | 5.6 | 53 |
| 1990 | 3 | 0.6 | 8.8 | 5.8 | 52 | 5.9 | 51 | 5.4 | 56 |
| 1991 | 2 | 0.2 | 7.3 | 6.4 | 31 | 6.3 | 32 | 6.6 | 30 |
| 1992 | 2 | 0.2 | 7.3 | 6.7 | 30 | 7.0 | 29 | 6.6 | 30 |
| 1993 | 10 | 4.8 | 18.4 | 7.4 | 136 | 7.3 | 138 | 7.7 | 130 |
| 1994 | 6 | 2.2 | 13.1 | 7.3 | 82 | 7.7 | 78 | 8.1 | 74 |
| 1995 | 15 | 8.4 | 24.8 | 7.8 | 192 | 7.9 | 190 | 8.1 | 185 |
| 1996 | 14 | 7.7 | 23.5 | 6.3 | 221 | 6.5 | 216 | 6.6 | 213 |
| 1997 | 11 | 5.5 | 19.7 | 4.9 | 227 | 4.9 | 222 | 4.8 | 227 |
| 1998 | 5 | 1.6 | 11.7 | 2.9 | 174 | 2.9 | 170 | 3.4 | 147 |

Table 9.7. Observed deaths among Shipman's male patients, 1987–1998, showing upper and lower 95% confidence limts. Table includes expected numbers of deaths based on estimates relating to England and Wales, manufacturing districts, and Tameside. SMR = standardised mortality rate among Shipman's patients; CL = confidence limit; Exp = expected.

| Males | All ages Observed | | | E&W standard | | Manufacturing standard | | Tameside standard | |
|---|---|---|---|---|---|---|---|---|---|
| | deaths | Lower CL | Upper CL | Exp | SMR | Exp | SMR | Exp | SMR |
| All years | 221 | 192.8 | 252.1 | 200.2 | 110 | 216.8 | 102 | 233.4 | 95 |
| 1987 | 21 | 13.0 | 32.1 | 14.3 | 147 | 14.1 | 149 | 17.2 | 122 |
| 1988 | 11 | 5.4 | 19.7 | 17.7 | 62 | 17.7 | 62 | 20.2 | 54 |
| 1989 | 22 | 13.7 | 33.3 | 17.8 | 124 | 17.9 | 123 | 20.2 | 109 |
| 1990 | 19 | 11.4 | 29.7 | 17.4 | 109 | 18.0 | 105 | 20.5 | 93 |
| 1991 | 16 | 9.1 | 26.0 | 17.5 | 91 | 18.4 | 87 | 19.2 | 83 |
| 1992 | 12 | 6.1 | 21.0 | 17.6 | 68 | 19.2 | 63 | 19.9 | 60 |
| 1993 | 19 | 11.4 | 29.7 | 18.8 | 101 | 20.0 | 95 | 20.8 | 92 |
| 1994 | 19 | 11.4 | 29.7 | 17.8 | 107 | 20.0 | 95 | 20.1 | 95 |
| 1995 | 26 | 16.9 | 38.1 | 17.6 | 148 | 19.6 | 132 | 22.1 | 118 |
| 1996 | 23 | 14.5 | 34.5 | 16.7 | 138 | 19.3 | 119 | 20.3 | 114 |
| 1997 | 20 | 12.2 | 30.9 | 15.8 | 126 | 18.9 | 106 | 18.9 | 106 |
| 1998 | 13 | 6.9 | 22.3 | 11.2 | 116 | 13.5 | 96 | 14.2 | 92 |

Table 9.8. Observed deaths among Shipman's male patients aged under 45, 1987–1998, showing upper and lower 95% confidence limits. Table includes expected numbers of deaths based on estimates relating to England and Wales, manufacturing districts, and Tameside. SMR = standardised mortality rate among Shipman's patients; CL = confidence limit; Exp = expected.

| Males | Under 45 Observed | | | E&W standard | | Manufacturing standard | | Tameside standard | |
|---|---|---|---|---|---|---|---|---|---|
| | deaths | Lower CL | Upper CL | Exp | SMR | Exp | SMR | Exp | SMR |
| All years | 15 | 8.3 | 24.8 | 17.2 | 87 | 18.6 | 81 | 19 | 79 |
| 1987 | 0 | 0.0 | 3.7 | 1.3 | 0 | 1.4 | 0 | 1.5 | 0 |
| 1988 | 1 | 0.0 | 5.6 | 1.6 | 61 | 1.7 | 59 | 1.6 | 62 |
| 1989 | 2 | 0.2 | 7.3 | 1.6 | 125 | 1.7 | 120 | 1.6 | 124 |
| 1990 | 1 | 0.0 | 5.6 | 1.7 | 59 | 1.7 | 58 | 1.7 | 59 |
| 1991 | 1 | 0.0 | 5.6 | 1.6 | 62 | 1.7 | 58 | 1.6 | 61 |
| 1992 | 1 | 0.0 | 5.6 | 1.5 | 66 | 1.7 | 60 | 1.7 | 59 |
| 1993 | 0 | 0.0 | 3.7 | 1.4 | 0 | 1.6 | 0 | 1.8 | 0 |
| 1994 | 1 | 0.0 | 5.6 | 1.4 | 71 | 1.6 | 64 | 1.4 | 73 |
| 1995 | 2 | 0.2 | 7.3 | 1.4 | 143 | 1.5 | 129 | 1.8 | 109 |
| 1996 | 4 | 1.1 | 10.3 | 1.4 | 286 | 1.6 | 255 | 1.6 | 243 |
| 1997 | 2 | 0.2 | 7.3 | 1.3 | 155 | 1.5 | 136 | 1.5 | 134 |
| 1998 | 0 | 0.0 | 3.7 | 0.9 | 0 | 1.0 | 0 | 1.2 | 0 |

Table 9.9. Observed deaths among Shipman's male patients aged 45–64, 1987–1998, showing upper and lower 95% confidence limits. Table includes expected numbers of deaths based on estimates relating to England and Wales, manufacturing districts, and Tameside. SMR = standardised mortality rate among Shipman's patients; CL = confidence limit; Exp = expected.

| Males 45–64 | Observed deaths | Lower CL | Upper CL | E&W standard Exp | SMR | Manufacturing standard Exp | SMR | Tameside standard Exp | SMR |
|---|---|---|---|---|---|---|---|---|---|
| All years | 50 | 37.1 | 65.9 | 38.5 | 130 | 44.2 | 113 | 47.0 | 106 |
| 1987 | 5 | 0.2 | 11.7 | 2.8 | 176 | 2.8 | 181 | 3.8 | 133 |
| 1988 | 4 | 1.1 | 10.3 | 3.3 | 120 | 3.3 | 121 | 4.0 | 100 |
| 1989 | 3 | 0.6 | 8.8 | 3.2 | 93 | 3.3 | 90 | 3.4 | 88 |
| 1990 | 6 | 2.2 | 13.1 | 3.3 | 183 | 3.5 | 172 | 4.2 | 142 |
| 1991 | 8 | 0.2 | 15.8 | 3.3 | 244 | 3.6 | 222 | 3.8 | 212 |
| 1992 | 2 | 0.2 | 7.3 | 3.3 | 60 | 3.8 | 53 | 3.7 | 53 |
| 1993 | 4 | 1.1 | 10.3 | 3.3 | 120 | 3.8 | 105 | 4.0 | 100 |
| 1994 | 5 | 1.6 | 11.7 | 3.3 | 153 | 4.0 | 125 | 4.0 | 124 |
| 1995 | 3 | 0.6 | 8.8 | 3.4 | 89 | 4.1 | 73 | 4.1 | 72 |
| 1996 | 3 | 0.6 | 8.8 | 3.4 | 87 | 4.3 | 69 | 4.1 | 73 |
| 1997 | 3 | 0.6 | 8.8 | 3.4 | 88 | 4.5 | 67 | 4.4 | 68 |
| 1998 | 4 | 1.1 | 10.3 | 2.4 | 164 | 3.2 | 124 | 3.3 | 119 |

Table 9.10. Observed deaths among Shipman's male patients aged 65–74, 1987–1998, showing upper and lower 95% confidence limits. Table includes expected numbers of deaths based on estimates relating to England and Wales, manufacturing districts, and Tameside. SMR = standardised mortality rate among Shipman's patients; CL = confidence limit; Exp = expected.

| Males 65–74 | Observed deaths | Lower CL | Upper CL | E&W standard Exp | SMR | Manufacturing standard Exp | SMR | Tameside standard Exp | SMR |
|---|---|---|---|---|---|---|---|---|---|
| All years | 48 | 35.4 | 63.7 | 50.8 | 94 | 55.7 | 86 | 63.1 | 76 |
| 1987 | 6 | 2.2 | 13.1 | 4.3 | 139 | 4.3 | 141 | 5.4 | 110 |
| 1988 | 2 | 0.2 | 7.3 | 4.7 | 43 | 4.7 | 43 | 5.9 | 34 |
| 1989 | 7 | 2.8 | 14.5 | 4.6 | 154 | 4.6 | 152 | 5.8 | 122 |
| 1990 | 2 | 0.2 | 7.3 | 4.4 | 46 | 4.5 | 44 | 5.5 | 36 |
| 1991 | 3 | 0.6 | 8.8 | 4.5 | 67 | 4.8 | 63 | 5.0 | 60 |
| 1992 | 2 | 0.2 | 7.3 | 4.7 | 42 | 5.2 | 39 | 5.5 | 36 |
| 1993 | 7 | 2.8 | 14.5 | 5.1 | 137 | 5.5 | 126 | 6.3 | 112 |
| 1994 | 5 | 1.6 | 11.7 | 4.7 | 106 | 5.4 | 93 | 5.9 | 85 |
| 1995 | 4 | 1.1 | 10.3 | 4.1 | 98 | 4.7 | 86 | 5.5 | 73 |
| 1996 | 4 | 1.1 | 10.3 | 3.7 | 107 | 4.4 | 90 | 4.6 | 88 |
| 1997 | 4 | 1.1 | 10.3 | 3.5 | 115 | 4.3 | 93 | 4.4 | 91 |
| 1998 | 2 | 0.2 | 7.3 | 2.6 | 76 | 3.3 | 60 | 3.4 | 59 |

Table 9.11. Observed deaths among Shipman's male patients aged 75–84, 1987–1998, showing upper and lower 95% confidence limits. Table includes expected numbers of deaths based on estimates relating to England and Wales, manufacturing districts, and Tameside. SMR = standardised mortality rate among Shipman's patients; CL = confidence limit; Exp = expected.

| Males 75–84 | Observed deaths | Lower CL | Upper CL | E&W standard | | Manufacturing standard | | Tameside standard | |
|---|---|---|---|---|---|---|---|---|---|
| | | | | Exp | SMR | Exp | SMR | Exp | SMR |
| All years | 75 | 59.0 | 94.0 | 65.6 | 114 | 69.9 | 107 | 76.4 | 98 |
| 1987 | 8 | 3.5 | 15.8 | 4.8 | 167 | 4.8 | 168 | 5.5 | 145 |
| 1988 | 2 | 0.2 | 7.3 | 6.5 | 31 | 6.5 | 31 | 7.1 | 28 |
| 1989 | 6 | 2.2 | 13.1 | 6.5 | 92 | 6.5 | 92 | 7.6 | 79 |
| 1990 | 8 | 3.5 | 15.8 | 6.3 | 127 | 6.5 | 123 | 7.2 | 111 |
| 1991 | 3 | 0.6 | 8.8 | 6.1 | 49 | 6.4 | 47 | 6.8 | 44 |
| 1992 | 6 | 2.2 | 13.1 | 5.6 | 108 | 6.0 | 100 | 6.5 | 93 |
| 1993 | 6 | 2.2 | 13.1 | 5.3 | 114 | 5.5 | 109 | 5.5 | 109 |
| 1994 | 3 | 0.6 | 8.8 | 4.9 | 61 | 5.4 | 55 | 5.5 | 54 |
| 1995 | 10 | 4.8 | 18.4 | 5.6 | 178 | 6.1 | 163 | 7.6 | 131 |
| 1996 | 8 | 3.5 | 15.8 | 5.4 | 147 | 6.2 | 129 | 7.2 | 111 |
| 1997 | 10 | 4.8 | 18.4 | 5.2 | 192 | 6.1 | 163 | 5.8 | 173 |
| 1998 | 5 | 1.6 | 11.7 | 3.3 | 151 | 3.9 | 127 | 4.1 | 122 |

Table 9.12. Observed deaths among Shipman's male patients aged 85 and over, 1987–1998, showing upper and lower 95% confidence limits. Table includes expected numbers of deaths based on estimates relating to England and Wales, manufacturing districts, and Tameside. SMR = standardised mortality rate among Shipman's patients; CL = confidence limit; Exp = expected.

| Males 85 and over | Observed deaths | Lower CL | Upper CL | E&W standard | | Manufacturing standard | | Tameside standard | |
|---|---|---|---|---|---|---|---|---|---|
| | | | | Exp | SMR | Exp | SMR | Exp | SMR |
| All years | 33 | 22.7 | 46.4 | 28.0 | 118 | 28.3 | 116 | 27.9 | 118 |
| 1987 | 2 | 0.2 | 7.3 | 1.0 | 200 | 1.0 | 202 | 1.0 | 203 |
| 1988 | 2 | 0.2 | 7.3 | 1.6 | 124 | 1.6 | 126 | 1.7 | 120 |
| 1989 | 4 | 1.1 | 10.3 | 1.9 | 214 | 1.8 | 224 | 1.8 | 222 |
| 1990 | 2 | 0.2 | 7.3 | 1.8 | 111 | 1.8 | 112 | 1.8 | 109 |
| 1991 | 1 | 0.0 | 5.6 | 2.0 | 49 | 2.0 | 50 | 1.9 | 52 |
| 1992 | 1 | 0.0 | 5.6 | 2.5 | 40 | 2.6 | 39 | 2.4 | 41 |
| 1993 | 2 | 0.2 | 7.3 | 3.6 | 55 | 3.6 | 56 | 3.2 | 63 |
| 1994 | 5 | 1.6 | 11.7 | 3.4 | 147 | 3.6 | 140 | 3.2 | 154 |
| 1995 | 7 | 2.8 | 14.5 | 3.1 | 223 | 3.2 | 221 | 3.0 | 234 |
| 1996 | 4 | 1.1 | 10.3 | 2.7 | 149 | 2.8 | 144 | 2.8 | 145 |
| 1997 | 1 | 0.0 | 5.6 | 2.5 | 40 | 2.6 | 39 | 2.9 | 35 |
| 1998 | 2 | 0.2 | 7.3 | 1.9 | 107 | 2.0 | 101 | 2.2 | 93 |

The findings do confirm an excess number of deaths among Shipman's patients, in particular among older women. However, the excess is not as substantial as that indicated by review of records and cremation forms, or the analysis of MCCDs. Of 255 cases in which the patient died between 1987–1998 and records and/or cremation forms had survived, 151 (59.2%) were classified as highly suspicious and 38 (14.9%) as moderately suspicious (see Table 8.17). Thus, 189 were judged to be suspicious to some degree. The excess numbers of MCCDs issued by Shipman from 1987 to1998 relating to deaths irrespective of place of death was 201 (Table 9.13). Therefore, the findings from a review of records and cremation forms and inspection of MCCDs point to similar conclusions.

Table 9.13. The annual numbers of deaths among Shipman's patients identified in the prospective audit and the numbers of MCCDs issued by Shipman, showing the % of deaths each year for which Shipman issued MCCDs and the total number of excess MCCDs per year, calculated from Tables 8.15–8.20.

| Year | Deaths identified in the prospective audit | MCCDs issued by Shipman | % of total deaths for which Shipman issued MCCDs | Excess numbers of MCCDs |
|---|---|---|---|---|
| 1987 | 46 | 16 | 34.8 | 7.36 |
| 1988 | 44 | 19 | 43.2 | 10.31 |
| 1989 | 40 | 15 | 37.5 | 9.64 |
| 1990 | 36 | 8 | 22.2 | 3.62 |
| 1991 | 30 | 10 | 33.3 | 6.22 |
| 1992 | 25 | 6 | 24.0 | -0.16 |
| 1993 | 53 | 28 | 52.8 | 22.28 |
| 1994 | 38 | 14 | 36.8 | 9.39 |
| 1995 | 69 | 37 | 53.6 | 33.81 |
| 1996 | 66 | 41 | 65.1 | 35.73 |
| 1997 | 72 | 47 | 65.3 | 41.67 |
| 1998 | 43 | 24 | 55.8 | 21.56 |
| totals | 562 | 265 | 50.4 | 201.43 |

One potential explanation for the different findings obtained from the prospective analysis of all deaths is that the method is insufficiently sensitive to detect variations in the annual numbers of MCCDs issued by general practitioners themselves (Frankel et al, 2000). In the prospective audit, 265 MCCDs issued by Shipman were identified, 50.4% of the 526 deaths among his patients from 1987. As Table 9.13 shows, the proportion of deaths for which Shipman issued MCCDs varied from year to year and exceeded 50% in 1993 and from 1995 to 1998. In England and Wales in 1996, 54.5% of deaths occurred in NHS hospitals, 10.4% in non-NHS hospitals, 3.6% in a hospice and 2.9% elsewhere. Only 20% occurred in the patient's own home and 8.0% in other community established such as residential homes (Devis and Rooney, 1999). Table 9.14 shows the annual percentage of deaths certified by doctors that did not occur in hospitals or nursing homes. If the percentage of 8% given by Devis and Rooney (1999) for deaths in community establishments is taken as applying to deaths in nursing homes, it can be concluded that general practitioners issued, between 1987 and 1998, MCCDs for around 28–30% of deaths among their patients. Shipman only issued MCCDs for this proportion of his patients who died in 1990 and 1992 (Table 9.13).

Table 9.14. Percentage of deaths certified by doctors, for deaths that did not occur in hospitals/ nursing homes; England and Wales

| Year of Death | | Age at death | | | | |
|---|---|---|---|---|---|---|
| | All ages | <45 | 45-64 | 65-74 | 75-84 | 85+ |
| 1987 | 22 | 9 | 21 | 21 | 21 | 30 |
| 1988 | 22 | 9 | 20 | 21 | 21 | 29 |
| 1989 | 22 | 9 | 20 | 21 | 21 | 29 |
| 1990 | 22 | 9 | 21 | 21 | 21 | 29 |
| 1991 | 22 | 9 | 21 | 21 | 21 | 29 |
| 1992 | 22 | 9 | 20 | 20 | 20 | 28 |
| 1993 | 22 | 10 | 21 | 21 | 21 | 29 |
| 1994 | 22 | 10 | 20 | 20 | 20 | 28 |
| 1995 | 21 | 9 | 19 | 19 | 19 | 27 |
| 1996 | 20 | 9 | 18 | 18 | 19 | 26 |
| 1997 | 20 | 8 | 17 | 18 | 19 | 26 |
| 1998 | 19 | 8 | 17 | 17 | 18 | 25 |

**Table 9.15. Numbers of deaths among Shipman's patients certified by him, by year and age/sex group.**

| Certified by | Year of death | | | | | | | | | | | | |
|---|---|---|---|---|---|---|---|---|---|---|---|---|---|
| | 1987 | 1988 | 1989 | 1990 | 1991 | 1992 | 1993 | 1994 | 1995 | 1996 | 1997 | 1998 | 1987–1998 |
| **Shipman** | | | | | | | | | | | | | |
| **Persons** Approx. age | | | | | | | | | | | | | |
| 85+ | 1.5 | 10.5 | 1.5 | 0 | 1 | 2 | 9.5 | 4 | 11 | 9 | 7 | 4 | 61 |
| 75–84 | 10.5 | 5.5 | 9 | 2.5 | 6 | 1 | 10.5 | 3.5 | 10 | 22 | 23 | 9.5 | 113 |
| 65–74 | 3 | 2 | 4.5 | 1.5 | 1 | 2 | 5 | 2.5 | 12.5 | 5 | 12 | 8 | 59 |
| 45–64 | 1 | 1 | 0 | 4 | 2 | 0.5 | 3 | 4 | 2.5 | 4 | 5 | 2.5 | 29.5 |
| <45 | 0 | 0 | 0 | 0 | 0 | 0.5 | 0 | 0 | 1 | 1 | 0 | 0 | 2.5 |
| All ages | 16 | 19 | 15 | 8 | 10 | 6 | 28 | 14 | 37 | 41 | 47 | 24 | 265 |
| **Females** | | | | | | | | | | | | | |
| 85+ | 1 | 8.5 | 1 | 0 | 1 | 2 | 8.5 | 4 | 8 | 6.5 | 6 | 3.5 | 50 |
| 75–84 | 8 | 4.5 | 6.5 | 2.5 | 5 | 1 | 7.5 | 3.5 | 4.5 | 15.5 | 20 | 8 | 86.5 |
| 65–74 | 2 | 1 | 1.5 | 1.5 | 0 | 1 | 3 | 1.5 | 9 | 3 | 10 | 8 | 41.5 |
| 45–64 | 0 | 1 | 0 | 2 | 0 | 0 | 2 | 1 | 1.5 | 3 | 4 | 2.5 | 17 |
| <45 | 0 | 0 | 0 | 0 | 0 | 0 | 0 | 0 | 0 | 0 | 0 | 0 | 0 |
| All ages | 11 | 15 | 9 | 6 | 6 | 4 | 21 | 10 | 23 | 28 | 40 | 22 | 195 |
| **Males** | | | | | | | | | | | | | |
| 85+ | 0.5 | 2 | 0.5 | 0 | 0 | 0 | 1 | 0 | 3 | 2.5 | 1 | 0.5 | 11 |
| 75–84 | 2.5 | 1 | 2.5 | 0 | 1 | 0 | 3 | 0 | 5.5 | 6.5 | 3 | 1.5 | 26.5 |
| 65–74 | 1 | 1 | 3 | 0 | 1 | 1 | 2 | 1 | 3.5 | 2 | 2 | 0 | 17.5 |
| 45–64 | 1 | 0 | 0 | 2 | 2 | 0.5 | 1 | 3 | 1 | 1 | 1 | 0 | 12.5 |
| <45 | 0 | 0 | 0 | 0 | 0 | 0.5 | 0 | 0 | 1 | 1 | 0 | 0 | 2.5 |
| All ages | 5 | 4 | 6 | 2 | 4 | 2 | 7 | 4 | 14 | 13 | 7 | 2 | 70 |

**Table 9.16. Numbers of deaths among Shipman's patients certified by doctors other than him, by year and by age sex/group.**

| Certified by | Year of death | | | | | | | | | | | | |
|---|---|---|---|---|---|---|---|---|---|---|---|---|---|
| | 1987 | 1988 | 1989 | 1990 | 1991 | 1992 | 1993 | 1994 | 1995 | 1996 | 1997 | 1998 | 1987–1998 |
| **Others** | | | | | | | | | | | | | |
| Approx. age | | | | | | | | | | | | | |
| 85+ | 4.5 | 5.5 | 4.5 | 5 | 2 | 1 | 5 | 7 | 12.5 | 8.5 | 5 | 4 | 64.5 |
| 75–84 | 12 | 8 | 9.5 | 9 | 5.5 | 11 | 9.5 | 5 | 5.5 | 4.5 | 10 | 12.5 | 102 |
| 65–74 | 7.5 | 4.5 | 5 | 8 | 4.5 | 4 | 5.5 | 7 | 5.5 | 3.5 | 3 | 4.5 | 62.5 |
| 45–64 | 6 | 6 | 4 | 5 | 7 | 3 | 4 | 4 | 4.5 | 5.5 | 4 | 7 | 60 |
| <45 | 0 | 1 | 2 | 1 | 1 | 0 | 1 | 1 | 4 | 3 | 3 | 1 | 18 |
| All ages | 30 | 25 | 25 | 28 | 20 | 19 | 25 | 24 | 32 | 25 | 25 | 29 | 307 |
| **Females** | | | | | | | | | | | | | |
| Approx. age | | | | | | | | | | | | | |
| 85+ | 3 | 5.5 | 2 | 3 | 1 | 0 | 3.5 | 2 | 8.5 | 6.5 | 5 | 2 | 42 |
| 75–84 | 5.5 | 7 | 5 | 1 | 3.5 | 5 | 6.5 | 2 | 1.5 | 3.5 | 3 | 7.5 | 51 |
| 65–74 | 3.5 | 3.5 | 1 | 6 | 2.5 | 3 | 1 | 3 | 4.5 | 2 | 1 | 2.5 | 33.5 |
| 45–64 | 2 | 2 | 1 | 1 | 1 | 1 | 1 | 2 | 2.5 | 3 | 2 | 2 | 20.5 |
| <45 | 0 | 0 | 0 | 0 | 0 | 0 | 1 | 0 | 3 | 0 | 1 | 0 | 5 |
| All ages | 14 | 18 | 9 | 11 | 8 | 9 | 13 | 9 | 20 | 15 | 12 | 14 | 152 |
| **Males** | | | | | | | | | | | | | |
| Approx. age | | | | | | | | | | | | | |
| 85+ | 1.5 | 0 | 2.5 | 2 | 1 | 1 | 1.5 | 5 | 4 | 2 | 0 | 2 | 22.5 |
| 75–84 | 6.5 | 1 | 4.5 | 8 | 2 | 6 | 3 | 3 | 4 | 1 | 7 | 5 | 51 |
| 65–74 | 4 | 1 | 4 | 2 | 2 | 1 | 4.5 | 4 | 1 | 1.5 | 2 | 2 | 29 |
| 45–64 | 4 | 4 | 3 | 4 | 6 | 2 | 3 | 2 | 2 | 2.5 | 2 | 5 | 39.5 |
| <45 | 0 | 1 | 2 | 1 | 1 | 0 | 0 | 1 | 1 | 3 | 2 | 1 | 13 |
| All ages | 16 | 7 | 16 | 17 | 12 | 10 | 12 | 15 | 12 | 10 | 13 | 15 | 155 |

**Table 9.17. All deaths among Shipman's registered patients, whether certified by Shipman or another doctor.**

| All deaths | Year of death | | | | | | | | | | | | |
|---|---|---|---|---|---|---|---|---|---|---|---|---|---|
| | 1987 | 1988 | 1989 | 1990 | 1991 | 1992 | 1993 | 1994 | 1995 | 1996 | 1997 | 1998 | 1987–1998 |
| **Approx. age** | | | | | | | | | | | | | |
| 85+ | 6 | 16 | 6 | 5 | 3 | 3 | 14.5 | 11 | 23.5 | 17.5 | 12 | 8 | 125.5 |
| 75–84 | 22.5 | 13.5 | 18.5 | 11.5 | 11.5 | 12 | 20 | 8.5 | 15.5 | 26.5 | 33 | 22 | 215 |
| 65–74 | 10.5 | 6.5 | 9.5 | 9.5 | 5.5 | 6 | 10.5 | 9.5 | 18 | 8.5 | 15 | 12.5 | 121.5 |
| 45–64 | 7 | 7 | 4 | 9 | 9 | 3.5 | 7 | 8 | 7 | 9.5 | 9 | 9.5 | 89.5 |
| <45 | 0 | 1 | 2 | 1 | 1 | 0.5 | 1 | 1 | 5 | 4 | 3 | 1 | 20.5 |
| All ages | 46 | 44 | 40 | 36 | 30 | 25 | 53 | 38 | 69 | 66 | 72 | 53 | 572 |
| **Females** | | | | | YoD | | | | | | | | |
| **Approx. age** | | | | | | | | | | | | | |
| 85+ | 4 | 14 | 3 | 3 | 2 | 2 | 12 | 6 | 16.5 | 13 | 11 | 5.5 | 92 |
| 75–84 | 13.5 | 11.5 | 11.5 | 3.5 | 8.5 | 6 | 14 | 5.5 | 6 | 19 | 23 | 15.5 | 137.5 |
| 65–74 | 5.5 | 4.5 | 2.5 | 7.5 | 2.5 | 4 | 4 | 4.5 | 13.5 | 5 | 11 | 10.5 | 75 |
| 45–64 | 2 | 3 | 1 | 3 | 1 | 1 | 3 | 3 | 4 | 6 | 6 | 4.5 | 37.5 |
| <45 | 0 | 0 | 0 | 0 | 0 | 0 | 1 | 0 | 3 | 0 | 1 | 0 | 5 |
| All ages | 25 | 33 | 18 | 17 | 14 | 13 | 34 | 19 | 43 | 43 | 52 | 36 | 347 |
| **Males** | | | | | | | | | | | | | |
| **Approx. age** | | | | | | | | | | | | | |
| 85+ | 2 | 2 | 3 | 2 | 1 | 1 | 2.5 | 5 | 7 | 4.5 | 1 | 2.5 | 33.5 |
| 75–84 | 9 | 2 | 7 | 8 | 3 | 6 | 6 | 3 | 9.5 | 7.5 | 10 | 6.5 | 77.5 |
| 65–74 | 5 | 2 | 7 | 2 | 3 | 2 | 6.5 | 5 | 4.5 | 3.5 | 4 | 2 | 46.5 |
| 45–64 | 5 | 4 | 3 | 6 | 8 | 2.5 | 4 | 5 | 3 | 3.5 | 3 | 5 | 52 |
| <45 | 0 | 1 | 2 | 1 | 1 | 0.5 | 0 | 1 | 2 | 4 | 2 | 1 | 15.5 |
| All ages | 21 | 11 | 22 | 19 | 16 | 12 | 19 | 19 | 26 | 23 | 20 | 17 | 225 |

**Table 9.18. Percentage of all deaths among Shipman's patients that were certified by him, by year and age/sex groups.**

| Percentage of deaths | Year of death | | | | | | | | | | | | |
|---|---|---|---|---|---|---|---|---|---|---|---|---|---|
| | 1987 | 1988 | 1989 | 1990 | 1991 | 1992 | 1993 | 1994 | 1995 | 1996 | 1997 | 1998 | 1987–1998 |
| **Certified by Shipman** | | | | | | | | | | | | | |
| **Approx. age** | | | | | | | | | | | | | |
| 85+ | 25 | 66 | 25 | 0 | 33 | 67 | 66 | 36 | 47 | 51 | 58 | 50 | 49 |
| 75–84 | 47 | 41 | 49 | 22 | 52 | 8 | 53 | 41 | 65 | 83 | 70 | 43 | 53 |
| 65–74 | 29 | 31 | 47 | 16 | 18 | 33 | 48 | 26 | 69 | 59 | 80 | 64 | 49 |
| 45–64 | 14 | 14 | 0 | 44 | 22 | 14 | 43 | 50 | 36 | 42 | 56 | 26 | 33 |
| <45 | 0 | 0 | 0 | 0 | 100 | 0 | 0 | 20 | 25 | 0 | 0 | 12 | |
| All ages | 35 | 43 | 38 | 22 | 33 | 24 | 53 | 37 | 54 | 62 | 65 | 45 | 46 |
| **Females** | | | | | | | | | | | | | |
| **Approx. age** | | | | | | | | | | | | | |
| 85+ | 25 | 61 | 33 | 0 | 50 | 100 | 71 | 67 | 48 | 50 | 55 | 64 | 54 |
| 75–84 | 59 | 39 | 57 | 71 | 59 | 17 | 54 | 64 | 75 | 82 | 87 | 52 | 63 |
| 65–74 | 36 | 22 | 60 | 20 | 0 | 25 | 75 | 33 | 67 | 60 | 91 | 76 | 55 |
| 45–64 | 0 | 33 | 0 | 67 | 0 | 0 | 67 | 33 | 38 | 50 | 67 | 56 | 45 |
| <45 | | | | 0 | | | | | | | | | |
| All ages | 44 | 45 | 50 | 35 | 43 | 31 | 62 | 53 | 53 | 65 | 77 | 61 | 56 |
| **Males** | | | | | | | | | | | | | |
| **Approx. age** | | | | | | | | | | | | | |
| 85+ | 25 | 100 | 17 | 0 | 0 | 0 | 40 | 0 | 43 | 56 | 100 | 20 | 33 |
| 75–84 | 28 | 50 | 36 | 0 | 33 | 0 | 50 | 0 | 58 | 87 | 30 | 23 | 34 |
| 65–74 | 20 | 50 | 43 | 0 | 33 | 50 | 31 | 20 | 78 | 57 | 50 | 0 | 38 |
| 45–64 | 20 | 0 | 0 | 33 | 25 | 20 | 25 | 60 | 33 | 29 | 33 | 0 | 24 |
| <45 | | | | 16 | | | | | | | | | |
| All ages | 24 | 36 | 27 | 11 | 25 | 17 | 37 | 21 | 54 | 57 | 35 | 12 | 31 |

Table 9.15 and 9.16 show the numbers of deaths among Shipman's patients certified by Shipman or other doctors respectively. Table 9.17 shows the total numbers of deaths among Shipman's patients, irrespective of who certified death. These data enable the percentages of deaths certified by Shipman himself to be calculated, and the findings are shown in Table 9.18.

Although it would have been expected that Shipman would have certified approximately 30% of all deaths himself, the percentage is higher in certain years in different age and sex groups. The difference is clearly evident from 1995 onwards among older women, but the findings also point to a difference among women in the 45-64 age group. Furthermore, differences are also suggested in other years. The percentage of deaths certified by Shipman himself is also raised among older males from 1995. In general, however, he certified the expected percentage of deaths among the younger age groups.

# 9.4 Conclusion

The prospective analysis has confirmed the finding of an excess number of deaths, particularly in older women. Among women of all ages, the excess was significantly greater than expected in 1988, 1993 and 1995 onwards. These findings support the findings of the analysis of MCCDs, and the reviews of clinical records and cremation forms. However, the total number of excess deaths was lower, and an excess was not identified among males.

An important factor in explaining these differences is that the prospective analysis included all deaths rather than only those certified by Shipman. Further analyses of the data have shown that Shipman issued a higher proportion of MCCDs himself among older women in all years other than 1992. The percentage was also high among older men in later years. These findings are compatible with the findings from the retrospective analysis of MCCDs issued by Shipman.

Another potential explanation for the different estimates of excess deaths is that the rates of death among the patients of the comparison practitioners was lower than that among Tameside in general. Nevertheless, since the Jarman and Townsend scores of the patients of Shipman and the comparison practitioners was similar (Section Three), Shipman would have been expected to have had similar rates to those of his local colleagues. The findings do not suggest that low numbers of patients died in hospital or other institutions (Table 9.16).

Thus, the prospective audit does not exclude the possibility that the excess detected in the analysis of MCCDs was, to some extent, an overestimate. Since the two methods of estimating the excess used different calculations, it is not surprising that the resulting numbers are different, The findings of the prospective audit produce generally lower figures until the later years, and there could be contributions due to chance or selection mechanisms because of Shipman's previous activities that may have had an impact on the size and characteristics of the population at risk. Even so, it is clear that in the later years, there was an excess of deaths whichever way the calculations are done.

The prospective audit has shown that the detection of an excess number of deaths among patients cared for in their terminal illnesses by Shipman would be more difficult using data about numbers of deaths in the population of registered patients. The method is insufficiently sensitive to identify relatively large excesses over a short period, or smaller excesses over a long period. Therefore, a system for monitoring death rates of general practitioners based only on deaths in registered populations cannot be recommended. However, prospective monitoring is necessary to ensure that conclusions are based on real excesses.

# Ten: Conclusions

## 10.1 Introduction

In this Section, general conclusions arising from the audit are presented. It must be emphasised, however, that the audit was concerned specifically with Shipman's clinical practice, and that the sources of evidence were various documents and records directly relating to the patient care (including prescribing) that he delivered or claimed to have delivered. The information that could have been provided by witnesses to Shipman's working life was deliberately excluded. The collection and evaluation of such information is more properly a matter for the Inquiry and the police. Although the audit did seek to describe factually the circumstances applying to the deaths of Shipman's patients, it cannot explain how or why the events came to happen. Furthermore, it cannot establish beyond doubt the cause of death of any individual patient or group of patients.

Various recording systems and registers have been reviewed in detail during the course of the audit. No recording system is perfect, however, and the extent to which reliance can be placed on the information contained therein must be a matter of judgement. Although it is conceivable that a very small number of MCCDs issued by Shipman and the comparison practitioners may have been overlooked, the numbers would have been too few to affect the conclusions. The check of cremation registers provides reassurance that almost all MCCDs issued by Shipman or the comparison practitioners in the earlier years had been identified.

Detailed information about the numbers and characteristics of the patients registered with Shipman was available only from 1987. The numbers and age/sex distribution prior to 1987 were estimated, but the effects of alternative assumptions were explored in two extreme scenarios. These analyses confirmed that the general conclusions remained stable despite the use of different assumptions about Shipman's list of patients.

Information about the circumstances of death was taken from surviving clinical records and cremation forms, and the findings provide support to the conclusions of the analysis of MCCDs. Records or cremation forms (or both) were available for 288 (89%) of all deaths for which Shipman issued MCCDs from 1985 onwards. Apart from a few surviving cremation forms, no information was available about the circumstances of deaths between 1974 and 1984. Therefore, inferences about events in these years rest solely on the brief details recorded on death notifications. It should also be recalled that it was established at the trial that Shipman had made false entries in clinical records and cremation forms in order to conceal his activities. In consequence, it may not have been possible to detect reasons for concern from some records.

The sources of information about the prescribing of restricted drugs were particularly inadequate. The pharmacies kept complete registers, sometimes for many years, but Shipman did not maintain a register, and the data collected by the Prescription Pricing Authority related only to a short period and do not permit the tracking of prescribing to individual patients.

# 10.2 Pattern of observed compared to expected deaths in particular age groups.

Care must be taken in making inferences from what can legitimately be quite large variations in mortality rates of patients of individual general practitioners (Frankel et al, 2000). Nevertheless, there is convincing evidence that the observed numbers of deaths among Shipman's patients was in excess of what would have been expected.

- Shipman issued a total of 521 MCCDs, 499 whilst he worked in Hyde. Over the same period, the highest number issued by a Hyde practitioner in the comparison group was 210.

- A comparison of the numbers of MCCDs issued by Shipman and a group of general practitioners with similar patients in the same locality in the same years indicated that he issued an excess total number of MCCDs of 297 (95% confidence interval 254 to 345), and an excess related to deaths at home of 236 (95% confidence interval 198 to 277).

- The review of clinical records and cremation forms suggests that the excess related to deaths at home (236) is most likely to reflect the true number of deaths about which there should be concern. Between 1985 and 1998, information from records and/or cremation forms was available for 288 (88.9%) of the 324 deaths for which Shipman issued MCCDs. 166 (57.6%) of these were classified as highly suspicious and 43 (14.9%) as moderately suspicious. The excess number of deaths among those dying at home between 1985 and 1998 was similar – 199.

- The excess varied between certain patient groups. The greatest excess was among females aged 75 or above, the second highest among females aged 65-74, and the third highest among males aged 75 or above. There was no excess among males aged below 65 years.

- The excess numbers became evident at an early stage of Shipman's career as a general practitioner. Among elderly females, the excess became apparent from his earliest years in practice.

- There was an excess of deaths in most years of Shipman's working life as a general practitioner.

- The excess was apparent among older women in the years preceding Shipman's arrest even in an analysis based on his population of registered patients rather than on MDDCs he issued himself.

- The prospective analysis of deaths among all Shipman's registered patients 1987–1998 indicated an excess of deaths among females in six of these 12 years, most consistently in those aged 75-84 and most evident from 1995.

Although evidence from records or cremation forms and MCCDs pointed to the same conclusion, the prospective analysis indicated a lower number of excess deaths. Whilst it is likely that the lower figure suggested in the prospective analysis is largely explained by the lack of ability of this method to detect even relatively large variations in the numbers of MCCDs issued by general practitioners, this different result should not be forgotten.

## 10.3 Deaths showing unusual clusters in time

There was a clear rise in the numbers of deaths towards the end of Shipman's career. The numbers of MCCDs issued by Shipman in these years reached levels several times greater than the numbers issued by the comparison practitioners. It is not surprising, therefore, that his activities eventually attracted attention. However, during 1998 a decline occurred in the numbers of MCCDs issued, at approximately the same time as the first investigation was initiated.

It should also be noted that death rates were low during Shipman's first year in the Todmorden practice and his first year in the Hyde group practice. The rates of deaths were generally higher than expected in most years of the 1980s, but between 1990–1992, the numbers of deaths were few. During this period, Shipman left the group practice and set up in practice alone.

There was also evidence of clusters of deaths in shorter periods of time. For example, deaths were more likely on certain weekdays. Occasionally several deaths would occur on the same day or within a few days, although this was not a frequent event. Information from cremation forms indicated that a higher proportion of Shipman's patients died in the afternoon in comparison with the patients of other Hyde general practitioners.

## 10.4 Deaths showing unusual clusters by place of death

A high proportion of deaths among Shipman's patients occurred at home and only one death in a residential home was classified as suspicious. It would have been difficult for Shipman to attend a patient in a residential or nursing home without a member of staff being in close attendance. Since staff would have been aware of the patient's general condition, it would have been difficult to explain unexpected deaths and, therefore, opportunities to administer lethal medication without fear of detection would have been limited. However, it would be unwise to assume that deaths in such accommodation were invariably natural.

A small number of deaths occurred in Shipman's practice premises. One death took place in the group practice in Hyde, and five in the single-handed practice. No deaths occurred in the practice premises in Todmorden. If patients of Shipman were excluded, the numbers of deaths on practice premises certified by general practitioners were very few. In the review of the coroner's files, one death occurring in a practice was identified, and post mortem confirmed natural causes. Referral of deaths on practice premises to a coroner would usually be the most appropriate course of action. However, it should be noted that only six of Shipman's patients died on practice premises, and this was not a common occurrence among deaths classified as suspicious.

## 10.5 The relationship between certified cause of death and medical history

At least some information about clinical history was available in records and cremation forms relating to 288 patients who died between 1985 and 1998. In these cases it was possible to relate elements of clinical history to certified cause of death, and the findings indicated that in a high proportion of cases, the association between history and cause of death was often tenuous. The history given by Shipman himself contributed to this problem but in other cases the history was not corroborated by the findings of other general practitioners or hospital doctors. In consequence of this and other factors, 166 cases were classified as highly suspicious and 43 as moderately suspicious.

The extent to which the weak relationship between clinical history and certified cause of death would have been evident from an inspection of a small number of records is uncertain. The review of a large number of records enabled the pattern to be clearly identified, but the records themselves were often very brief. Furthermore, it was established at the trial that Shipman had fabricated entries. Therefore, review of a small number of records without evidence of back-dated record entries could well have given rise to misleading conclusions.

# 10.6 The integrity of records

The records were poor. The legibility of hand written entries was often poor, and in both the paper and computer records, entries were generally brief and sometimes even perfunctory. Patient contacts were often not recorded on both systems, and it is likely that some contacts were recorded on neither system. Shipman did not appear to have a clear policy on when the paper or computer systems were to be used, and in consequence on many occasions there was no single clear account of patient care.

Shipman is known to have made false back-dated entries in his computer records, and additional examples were identified during the review. It was not possible to identify false entries made prior to October 1996 since the computer audit trail was not installed until then. Nor was it possible to satisfactorily judge the extent to which any entries in the paper records were fabrications. Nevertheless, the findings are cause for considerable concern about the quality and veracity of Shipman's records.

# 10.7 The prescribing of restricted drugs

It has been established that Shipman murdered his victims by injections of lethal doses of diamorphine. He did not maintain a controlled drugs register, although he did personally carry and administer diamorphine. A review of his prescribing of restricted drugs confirmed that he had signed prescriptions for single doses of diamorphine for several patients in 1993. However, convincing evidence of excess prescribing of diamorphine was not identified. Evidence had been presented to the trial to confirm that Shipman collected unused doses of diamorphine following the terminal care of patients in their own homes, but the possibility that he also obtained restricted drugs from other sources cannot be ruled out.

# 10.8 Supporting staff

Inevitably the audit did involve some interaction with local health services and other agencies, although no systematic assessment of the operation of local health care services was planned or conducted. Nevertheless, one issue became apparent during the course of the audit.

Local practitioners reported receiving relatively little support from professional organisations or elected leaders of the community, although the Health Authority had been supportive. In addition to having to cope with the pressure caused by the events in Hyde, and with the concerns of their patients and community in the aftermath, the practitioners had to face a degree of professional isolation. The provision of more support from professional organisations might have helped the practitioners when distressed, and also contributed to the creation of a culture in which learning from adverse events is given a higher priority.

The primary care team at The Surgery, 21, Market Street provided important assistance in aspects of the audit. Yet at that time they were themselves uncertain about their future, and were faced with confronting the truth of Shipman's activities. They did have some support, but it would have been helpful if a senior member of NHS management had visited them to hear about their experiences.

It is my understanding that until I visited the team in May 2000, no senior person had been to the practice to discuss the distressing sequence of events.

# 10.9 Summary conclusion

The audit has uncovered a substantial body of evidence from various sources that raises grave concerns about Shipman's activities throughout the 25 years he spent as a general practitioner:

- replication of the typical features relating to the deaths of patients for which Shipman was convicted:

    - a high proportion of deaths among older women

    - a high proportion of deaths occurring at home

    - a high proportion of deaths occurring in the afternoon

    - Shipman was present at death or had seen the patient shortly before death in a high number of cases

    - a high proportion of patients were certified as having died from heart problems, strokes or old age

    - the association between clinical history and certified cause of death was often weak

- identification of further evidence to indicate:

    - an excess number of MCCDs issued by Shipman, irrespective of place of death

    - an excess number of MCCDs issued relating to deaths at home

    - an excess number of deaths among older women registered with Shipman in comparison with local and national rates

    - the pattern of excess deaths among older women could be identified early in Shipman's career as a general practitioner

    - a high proportion of patients died suddenly

    - poor record keeping, including poor legibility, brief record entries, and no clear policy on the use of computer and paper records

    - an inadequate audit trail relating to the prescribing of controlled drugs.

# Eleven: Recommendations

## 11.1 Introduction

When the audit was originally planned and commissioned, it was not envisaged nor required that recommendations would be made. However, the nature of the findings and the process of inspection of the various sources of data have clarified a number of issues which make the presentation of recommendations mandatory. Nevertheless, it is important to qualify the basis for the recommendations. First, they are personal and do not represent the views of any group or institution. Second, they rest on limited sources of evidence and observations made during the course of the audit. Therefore, they should be regarded as starting points for further discussion on the steps that could be taken to prevent doctors such as Shipman murdering patients in the future.

## 11.2 Monitoring performance in general practice

Shipman did not undergo at any time during his career a review of his clinical performance that was sufficiently searching to uncover his activities. Indeed, it was not until he forged a will that an investigation uncovered evidence of murder. This points to a lack of accountability that is not acceptable.

The routine monitoring systems available to Health Authorities did not detect the extent of the problems, and since Shipman was not a general practice trainer he would not have undergone the regular inspections required for that post. Furthermore, since he was not a member of the Royal College of General Practitioners it is unlikely that he took part in any of the College's performance review schemes.

A series of major reforms is now being implemented to ensure improved monitoring and accountability of doctors, including:

- the introduction of clinical governance and the creation of the Commission for Health Improvement with powers to undertake regular inspections (Secretary of State for Health, 1997)

- regular revalidation of all doctors to ensure they demonstrate fitness to practise (GMC, 2000b)

- annual appraisal and a system to address poor performance (Department of Health, 1999)

- mechanisms to enable the health service to detect and learn from adverse events (Department of Health, 2000)

- plans for new contractual quality standards for single-handed practices and further development of the Personal Medical Services contract (Secretary of State for Health, 2000).

These developments are, however, designed to monitor and improve the performance of doctors and other health professionals rather than detect the murder of patients.

*Recommendation 1. Systems for the monitoring of general practitioners should be reviewed and extended to include routine monitoring of death rates, and improved methods for the review of prescribing of controlled drugs and the quality of medical records.*

# 11.3 Monitoring death rates

Health professionals who murder patients are rare, but not unknown. The most recent case in the UK was that of the nurse Beverly Allitt (Allitt Inquiry, 1994). In 1993, Allitt was convicted of the murder of four children, the attempted murder of three others, and grievous bodily harm of six more. In the United States, a doctor was convicted in September 2000 of the murder of three patients, but is suspected of murdering up to 60 (Woods, 2000). Health services must accept responsibility for protecting patients from such individuals. The public cannot be expected to have confidence in a system that fails to detect the murder of a large number of patients over a period of years by a doctor or other health professional.

It is clear from the audit that there is no system in place for monitoring death rates among patients of general practitioners. In the absence of such a system, it is possible for a general practitioner with a sustained excess rate of deaths to go undetected for many years. One difficulty in using of death rates among registered lists of patients to monitor general practitioners lies in the variability of rates. Substantial variation occurs even at the level of a primary are group (Majeed et al, 2000). Another difficulty is that general practitioners are not involved in the management of many of their patients who die. In 1996 in England and Wales, only 21% of all deaths occurred in the patient's own home and 8% occurred in residential and other community homes (Devis and Rooney, 1999). In consequence, a very high death rate in any one year would be required in order to trigger an investigation (Frankel et al, 2000).

The alternative suggested by Frankel and colleagues was 'strengthened avenues for informal intelligence of aberrant practice from patients, relatives, other doctors, practice staff, pharmacists, coroners, undertakers and others'. However, as the events leading up to Shipman's arrest show, it is extremely difficult for fellow general practitioners to detect abnormal death rates associated with a colleague. The audit has highlighted some factors that might improve the ability of monitoring systems to detect criminal activity. The monitoring of MCCDs issued by general practitioners rather than death rates among all their registered patients would be more sensitive to their clinical activities. Additional information including place of death, duration of terminal illness and persons present at death should be explored as approaches to improving the sensitivity and specificity of monitoring. The potential role of monitoring of cumulative excess death rates should also be investigated.

The collection of data is not in itself sufficient since a mechanism is also required for the regular review of the findings. Annual appraisal and periodic revalidation present opportunities for the discussion of death rates with general practitioners, but the potential advantages and disadvantages of such an approach must be considered in the context of the objectives of appraisal in particular. The arguments against the introduction of a monitoring system are that it would require the investment of time and other resources when general practitioners are already over stretched, and that it would be unnecessary since cases such as Shipman's are exceptionally rare and individuals determined on murder would adopt strategies to avoid detection.

There are feasible methods for collecting information about death rates in relation to general practitioners. The options include registers maintained by general practitioners themselves, or registers compiled from the Public Health Mortality File by Health Authorities. The system of Newcastle Health Authority is an example of the latter (Stacey et al, 1998). Examples of the former can be found in the work of several general practitioners (Berlin et al, 1993; Khunti, 1996; Khunti, 2000). These systems require development to ensure that MCCDs issued by general practitioners are distinguished from MCCDs issued by other doctors.

*Recommendation 2: A system for collecting information about the numbers of deaths of patients of, and MCCDs issued by, general practitioners should be investigated, and a practical system introduced as soon as possible.*

# 11.4 Death certification procedures

Since a review of death certification procedures is already being undertaken by the Home Office (www.homeoffice.gov.uk/ccpd/bkgrnd00.htm), detailed recommendations are not included in this report. However, the findings of the audit highlight the potential importance of corroborative evidence about the cause of death.

The practice of requiring a second doctor to confirm the circumstances of death prior to cremation (Form C) is of little value. However, Shipman himself provided a clue as to how the system could be improved. Corroborative information obtained from clinical records, other health professionals or relatives and carers offers an important resource in confirming the circumstances and cause of death. A routine requirement for corroborative evidence would have it made more difficult for Shipman to have avoided detection.

Cremation Form B records information about the circumstances of death, but MCCDs do not. Neither record details of the clinical history. In the audit, information about the circumstances of death greatly increased the ability of a fellow professional to make judgements about levels of suspicion.

*Recommendation 3: In a revised certification system, brief information about the circumstances of death and the patient's clinical history should be recorded both in the case of cremations and burials.*

# 11.5 General practice records

Shipman's records were extremely poor. The use of dual systems, neither of which contained a full account of patient care, served to obscure his activities and allow him to blame poor record keeping rather than fabrication for any inconsistencies. I am not aware of any previous review of Shipman's recording habits. It is clearly unacceptable that a practitioner should be allowed to maintain inadequate records without ever being required to address the problem. Practical and efficient methods for reviewing the quality of records are required.

Some of the deficiencies of Shipman's records arose from the use of dual record systems. There was no clear policy on the use of each system, and he waited until returning to the practice, sometimes the following day, before recording information about home visits. Shipman's computer entries were so brief as to be inadequate, and his records on paper were also brief. New regulations governing arrangements to allow general practitioners to maintain part or all of their patient records on computer were introduced from October 2000 (Statutory Instrument 2000 No 2383). The regulations also require general practitioners to keep adequate records.

*Recommendation 4: The procedure for revalidation of general practitioners should include an assessment of appropriate samples of a general practitioner's records.*

The discovery of clinical records of deceased patients in Shipman's home gives rise to another matter that should be considered.

*Recommendation 5: The policy of offering to return records to general practitioners after the expiry of the period of storage by Health Authorities should be reviewed. If general practitioners are allowed to retain records, arrangements for their secure storage should be established, and provision for their eventual disposal agreed.*

# 11.6 Controlled drugs

Shipman did not maintain a controlled drugs register. It is unacceptable that this state of affairs should have gone unnoticed and unchallenged, and improved arrangements for review of controlled drugs registers require review. Routine inspections used to be undertaken by the Medical Officers of the Regional Medical Service, but this arrangement was discontinued when the service was disbanded, and there appears to be confusion about who is now responsible for inspection.

One option could be to allow the Inspectors of the Royal Pharmaceutical Society to take on this function. The Society's Inspectors are thoroughly versed in relevant legislation and in techniques for encouraging improved practice. However, to extend their role to general practices would require an increase in the number of inspectors and adequate financial support. An alternative would be to include review of the controlled drugs register during appraisals and/or revalidation.

*Recommendation 6: An effective system for the inspection of general practitioners' controlled drugs registers should be introduced.*

Shipman did not record the batch number of controlled drugs that he administered to patients himself. Furthermore, neither pharmacies or general practitioners are required to record batch numbers of controlled drugs in their controlled drugs registers. The omission of batch numbers is a major weakness in constructing an audit trail for controlled drugs from requisition by a pharmacy to administration to a patient or disposal.

*Recommendation 7: General practitioners should record batch numbers in clinical records when they personally administer controlled drugs, and batch numbers should be included in the controlled drugs registers of general practitioners and pharmacists.*

# 11.7 Review of care of individual deceased patients

The review of Shipman's records and cremation forms disclosed a pattern that gave rise to considerable concern. It is possible, therefore, that review of individual cases may have revealed Shipman's activities at an earlier stage. Such reviews could be linked to appraisal or revalidation procedures, and cases could be selected from death registers or the Public Health Mortality File. However, there is little evidence to suggest how practical or effective such a system would be, and therefore it is not appropriate to make a recommendation. Nevertheless, the critical incident technique has been used in audit of deaths (Redpath et al, 1996; Berlin et al, 1992), and further research in this field should be encouraged.

# References

Allitt Inquiry (1994). *Independent inquiry relating to deaths and injuries on the children's ward at Grantham and Kesteven General Hospital during the period February to April 1991* (The Clothier Report). London: HMSO.

Bailey S, Charlton J, Dollamore J, Fitzpatrick J (2000). Families, groups and clusters of local and health authorities: revised for authorities in 1999. *Population Trends 99.* Spring 2000, 37–52.

Berlin A, Bhopal R, Spencer J, Van Zwanenberg T (1996). Creating a death register for general practice. *Br J Gen Pract 43*:70–2.

Berlin A, Spencer JA, Bhopal RS, van Zwanenberg TD (1992). Audit of deaths in general practice: pilot study of the critical incident technique. *Quality in Health Care* 1:231–235.

Cremation Society of Great Britain (1999). National Cremation Statistics, 1960–1997. http://members.aol.com/cremsoc/LegalEtc/Stats/StatsNat.html

Department of Health (1994). *Preservation, retention, and destruction of GP general medical services records relating to patients.* FHSL (94)30. Leeds.

Department of Health (1998). *Preservation, retention, and destruction of GP general medical services records relating to patients.* Health Service Circular. HSC 1998/217.

Department of Health (2000). *An organisation with a memory.* London: The Stationary Office.

Department of Health (1999). *Supporting doctors, protecting patients.* London: Department of Health.

Devis T, Rooney C (1999). Death certification and the epidemiologist. *Health Statistics Quarterly.* Spring, 21–33.

Frankel S, Sterne J, Smith GD (2000). Mortality variations are a measure of general practitioner performance: implications of the Shipman case. BMJ 320:489.

Gardner MJ, Altman DG (1989). *Statistics with Confidence.* London: BMJ.

General Medical Council (1995). *Good Medical Practice.* London: GMC.

General Medical Council (2000a). *Confidentiality: Protecting and Providing Information.* London: GMC, September 2000.

General Medical Council (2000b). *Revalidating Doctors. Ensuring standards, securing the future.* London: GMC.

General Medical Practice Computer Systems RFA V4 (1997). NHS Information Management Centre.

Jarman B (1985). Underprivileged areas. In: Gray DJP, editor. *The Medical Annual 1985.* Bristol: Wight. P224–243.

Joint Computing Group of the General Practitioners' Committee and the Royal College of General Practitioners (2000). *Good Practice Guidelines for General Practice Electronic Records.* London: Joint Computing Group.

Khunti K (1996). A method of creating a death register for general practice. *BMJ* 312:952.

Khunti K (2000). Referral for autopsies: analysis of 651 consecutive deaths in one general practice. *Post Grad Med J* 76:415–6.

Majeed A, Bardsley M, Morgan D, O'Sullivan C, Bindman AB (2000). (cross sectional study of primary care groups in London: association of measures of socio-economic and health status with hospital admission rates. *BMJ* 321:1057–60.

PPA (1994). *New PACT for GPs*. A distance learning pack for GPs. (with: National Medical Advisers Support Centre and Centre for Pharmacy Education). London: HMSO.

Redpath L, Stacey A, Pugh E, Holmes E (1997). Use of the critical incident technique in primary care audit of deaths by suicide. *Quality in Health Care* 6:25–28.

Secretary of State for Health (1997). *The new NHS Modern Dependable*. London: The Stationery Office Limited.

Secretary of State for Health (2000. *The NHS Plan*. London: The Stationery Office Limited.

Stacey R, Robinson L, Bhopal R, Spencer J (1998). Evaluation of death registers in general practice. *Br J Gen Pract* 48: 1739–41.

Statistical Bulletin (2000). Statistics for General Medical Practitioners in England: 1989–1999. Bulletin 2000/8.

Townsend P, Phillimore P, Beattie A (1988). *Health and Deprivation. Inequality and the North*. London: Croom Helm.

Woods D (2000). US doctor may have killed 60. *BMJ* 321:657.

# Appendix 1. A summary of the career of Harold Frederick Shipman

This summary was constructed from information from Greater Manchester Police, the Department of Health, and the 1996 medical register.

| | |
|---|---|
| Date of birth | 14/1/1946 |
| 1965–1970 | Leeds University Medical School |
| 1970 | Gained MBChB |
| 23 July 1970 | Provisional registration with GMC (Number 1470473) |
| 1 Aug 1970<br>31 Jan 1971 | Pre-registration house officer (surgery) Pontefract General Infirmary |
| 1 Feb 1971<br>31 July 1971 | Pre-registration house officer (medicine) Pontefract General Infirmary |
| 5 Aug 1971 | Full registration with GMC, number 1470473 |
| Sept 1972 | Diploma in Child Health (DCH) |
| Sept 1973 | Diploma of Royal College of Obstetricians and Gynaecologists (DRCOG); Number A9640 |
| 1 March 1974-<br>31 March 1974 | Assistant general practitioner, Todmorden Group Practice, Todmorden |
| 1 April 1974-<br>Sept 1975 | General practitioner principal, Todmorden Group Practice, Todmorden |
| 1976 | Convicted of dishonestly obtaining drugs, forgery of an NHS prescription, and unlawful possession of pethidine. He was fined on each charge and ordered to pay compensation to the local Family Practitioner Committee. These offences were reported to the GMC, who told Shipman that if he offended again, these cases would form part of a subsequent hearing. Medical reports at that time said that he was unlikely to offend again. |
| 11 Dec 1975 | Break in practice, 1 year and 294 days |
| 1977 | Clinical Medical Officer, South West Durham. His responsibilities are reported as having being limited to examination of infants and advice about development. |
| 1 Oct 1977<br>31 Dec 1991 | General practitioner principal, Donneybrook House Group Practice, Hyde |

| | |
|---|---|
| 1985 | The GMC received a complaint alleging that Shipman had provided inadequate medical care in a young man who died from an undiagnosed illness. The complaint was referred back to the Family Practitioner Committee. |
| 1989 | A complaint was made that Shipman had prescribed the wrong dose of Epilim to a patient with epilepsy. The complaint was upheld, but there was no withholding from his remuneration. A civil case for negligence was pursued and settled for £250,000. |
| 1 Jan 1992 31 May 1992 | General practitioner principal, Donneybrook House, Hyde, operating as a single-handed GP |
| 1992 | A complaint for failure to visit was upheld |
| 1 June 1992 | General practitioner principal, the Surgery, 21 Market Street, Hyde |
| 1995 | A complaint about inadequate/incorrect treatment was made but the patient did not pursue the complaint |
| 24 Mar 1998 | Concerns about excess number of deaths among Shipman's patients reported by local general practitioners to Stockport coroner |
| 7 Sept 1998 | Arrested by Greater Manchester Police |

# Appendix 2. Cremation Forms B and C as used at Dukinfield crematorium

DUKINFIELD CREMATORIUM
Telephone: 061-330 1901.

# Forms B C and D

## CREMATION ACTS, 1902 and 1952.

*Statutory Rules and Orders, 1930 and 1952.*

**These Forms are Statutory. All the questions must be answered therefore, to make the Certificate effective for the purpose of Cremation.**

**These medical certificates are regarded as strictly confidential. The right to inspect them is confined to the Secretary of State, the Ministry of Health and the Chief Officer of a Police Force.**

## Forms B

CERTIFICATE OF MEDICAL ATTENDANT.

**I am informed** that application is about to be made for the cremation of the remains of:

*(Name of Deceased)* ...............................................................................................................

*(Address)* ..........................................................................................................................

*(Occupation or Description)*........................................................................ *(Age)* ......................

**Having attended** the Deceased before death, and seen and identified the body after death, I give the following answers to the questions set out below:–

(1) This form is not to be used in the case of a Coroner's Inquest.

(2) NOTE – The answers to the questions should be as concise as possible. Figures may be used instead of words.

ALL the questions must be answered.

| | |
|---|---|
| 1. On what date and at what hour, did he or she die? | |
| 2. What was the place where the deceased died? (Give address and say whether own residence, lodging, hotel, hospital, nursing home, etc.) | |
| 3. Are you a relative of the deceased? If so, state the relationship. | |
| 4. Have you, so far as you are aware any pecuniary interest in the death of the deceased? | |
| 5. (a) Were you the ordinary medical attendant of the deceased? | (a)........................................................ |
|     (b) If so, for how long? | (b)........................................................ |
| 6. (a) Did you attend the deceased during his or her last illness? | (a)........................................................ |
|     (b) If so, for how long? | (b)........................................................ |
| 7. When did you last see the deceased alive? (Say how many days or hours before death.) | |
| | *(The doctor must see the body after death).* |
| 8. (a) How soon after death did you see the body? | (a)........................................................ |
|     (b) What examination of it did you make? | (b)........................................................ |

☞

SEE NOTE OVERLEAF.

| | |
|---|---|
| 8A. If the deceased died in a hospital* at which he was an in-patient, has a post-mortem examination been made by a registered medical practitioner of not less than five years' standing who is neither a relative of the deceased nor a relative or partner of yours and are the results of that examination known to you? | |

(3) If the death has been reported to Coroner for any reason, this should be stated in answer to question 18.

| | |
|---|---|
| 9. What was the cause of death? | |
| I | |
| Immediate cause. | (a) ........................................... |
| | due to |
| Morbid conditions, if any, giving rise to immediate cause (stated in order proceeding backwards from immediate cause). | (b) ........................................... |
| | due to |
| | (c) ........................................... |
| II | |
| Other morbid conditions (if important) contributing to death but not related to immediate cause. | ........................................... |

(OVER)

| | |
|---|---|
| 10. (a) What was the mode of death?<br>(Say whether syncope, coma, exhaustion, convulsions, etc.)<br>(b) What was its duration in days hours, or minutes? | (a).................................................................................<br><br>(b)................................................................................. |
| 11. State how far the answers to the last <u>two</u> questions are the result of your own observations, or are based on statements made by others.<br><br>If on statements made by others, say by whom. | |
| 12. (a) Did the deceased undergo any operation during the final illness or within a year before death?<br><br>(b) If so, what was its nature and who performed it? | (a)................................................................................<br><br>(b)................................................................................ |
| 13. By whom was the deceased nursed during his or her last illness?<br><br>(Give names and say whether professional nurse, relative, etc. If the illness was a long one this question should be answered with reference to the period of four weeks before the death). | |
| 14. Who were the persons (if any) present at the moment of death? | |
| 15. In view of the knowledge of the deceased's habits and constitution, do you feel any doubt whatever as to the character of the disease or the cause of death ? | |
| 16. Have you any reason to suspect, that the death of the deceased was due, directly or indirectly, to<br>(a) Violence  ...  ...  ...  ...  ...  ...<br>(b) Poison  ...  ...  ...  ...  ...  ...<br>(c) Privation or neglect  ...  ...  ... | *Death due directly or indirectly to alcohol has now to be reported to the Coroner.* |
| 17. Have you any reason whatever to suppose a further examination of the body to be desirable? | |
| 18. Have you given the certificate required for registration of death? If not who has? | |
| 19. Has the Coroner been notified?<br>if so please give **FULL DETAILS** | |

(4) When the certificate for registration has been given by authority of the Coroner, this fact should be stated.

**I Hereby Certify** that the answers given above are true and accurate to the best of my knowledge and belief, and that I know of no reasonable cause to suspect that the deceased died either violent or an unnatural death or a sudden death of which the cause is unknown or died in such place or circumstances as to require an inquest in pursuance of any Act.

*(Signature)* ....................................................................................

**NAME IN BLOCK CAPITALS PLEASE**    ...........................................    *(Address)*....................................................................................

*(Registered* Qualifications ............................................................

*(Date)* ...........................................*(Tel.)*........................................................

NOTE — *This certificate must be handed or sent in a closed envelope by the medical practitioner, who signs it, to the medical practitioner who is to give the confirmatory certificate below, "except in a case where question 8A overleaf is answered in the affirmative, in which case the certificate must be handed or sent to the Medical Referee".*

"*The term "hospital" as used here means any institution for the reception and treatment of persons suffering from illness or mental disorder, any maternity home, and any institution for the reception and treatment of persons during convalescence".

*Additional information regarding either of the Certificates may be given here if necessary*

Has a pacemaker or any radio active material been inserted in the deceased? (YES or NO).....................

If so, has it been removed? (YES or NO)....................

CREMATION CANNOT TAKE PLACE UNTIL IT HAS BEEN REMOVED.

# Form C

CONFIRMATORY MEDICAL CERTIFICATE

*Pursuant to No. 9 of the Cremation Regulations, 1930 and 1952.*

*The Confirmatory medical certificate in Form C, if not given by the Medical Referee must be given by a medical practitioner who has been registered in this country for not less than 5 years and who is not a relative of the deceased or a relative or partner of the doctor who has given the certificate in Form B.*

I, being neither a relative of the deceased, nor a relative or partner of the medical practitioner who has given the foregoing medical certificate, have examined it and have made personal inquiry as stated in any answers to the questions below:–

(5) Each question must be answered. The answers to Nos. (1), (2) & (4) should invariably be in the affirmative.

 See Note above

*The doctor must see the body of the deceased.*

1.  Have you seen the body of the deceased?

2.  Have you carefully examined the body externally?

3.  Have you made a post mortem examination?

4.  Have you seen and questioned the medical practitioner who gave the above certificate?

5.  (a)  Have you seen and questioned any other medical practitoner who attended the deceased?
    (b)  (Give names and addresses of persons seen and say whether you saw them alone.)

    (a) .............................................................
    (b) .............................................................

6.  (a)  Have you seen and questioned any person who nursed the deceased during his or her last illness, or who was present at the death?
    (b)  (Give names and addresses of persons seen and say whether you saw them alone.)

    (a) .............................................................
    (b) .............................................................

7.  (a)  Have you seen and questioned any of the relatives of the deceased?
    (b)  (Give names and addresses of persons seen and say whether you saw them alone.)

    (a) .............................................................
    (b) .............................................................

8.  (a)  Have you seen and questioned any other person?
    (b)  (Give names and addresses of persons seen and say whether you saw them alone.)

    (a) .............................................................
    (b) .............................................................

**I am satisfied** that the cause of death was ...........................................................

Here insert cause of death.

..................................................................................................................

and I certify that I know of no reasonable cause to suspect that the deceased died either a violent or an unnatural death or a sudden death of which the cause is unknown or died in such place of circumstances as to require an inquest in pursuance of any Act.

*(Signature)* ...........................................................

**NAME IN BLOCK CAPITALS PLEASE**

........................................................    *(Address)* ...........................................................

..................................................................................................................

*(Date)* ...........................................*(Tel.)*...........................................................

*Registered* Qualifications........................................................... *Year* ............
(One of which must be of 5 years standing as above).

*Appointment held* ...........................................................

NOTE –    These Certificates, after being signed by both medical men, must be handed or sent in a closed envelope to the **Registrar and Superintendent, Dukinfield Crematorium, Hall Green Road, Dukinfield,** by one or other of the Medical Practitioners by whom the Certificates are given. (Telephone: 061-330 1901).

Forms B & C must be delivered to the Crematorium not later than 11.00 a.m. on the day (exclusive of Sunday) before the Cremation. Any delay in the delivery of these forms may lead to a postponement of the Cremation.

# Appendix 3. Patterns of prescribing

## 1 Patterns of prescribing

A general review of Shipman's prescribing was undertaken to determine whether he was a typical prescriber in general, and whether they were any therapeutic areas in which his prescribing was atypical. Therapeutic areas of particular interest were drugs used in the treatment of cardiovascular disease, drugs used for mental disorders, and analgesics. The source of data was an electronic PACT file held by West Pennine Health Authority. In this file, data were available from January 1995, and the period of interest was therefore January 1995 to October 1998.

The Health Authority reported that Shipman's prescribing costs were consistently 60% above the Health Authority average. Improvements had not occurred following visits to the practice. The standard PACT report for the quarter ending September 1998 indicated that Shipman's costs were 73% above the Health Authority equivalent and 90% above the national equivalent.

A summary of Shipman's total costs in comparison with all other practices in Thameside is shown in Table A.1. The data include the total cost of prescriptions issued between January 1995 and October 1998, the total number of items, the percentage of items that were prescribed generically, the total cost per item, the total items per 1000 prescribing units and total cost per 1000 prescribing units. The prescribing unit (PU) chosen was the ASTRO unit, which provides a standardised means of comparing practices since the proportion of patients in different age groups is taken into account. Patients under 65 and temporary residents count as one PU. Patients aged 65 or over count as three.

Table A.1 shows that Shipman was an outlier in terms of prescribing costs. His total cost per item was almost £3.00 more than any other practice in the group. The total cost per 1000 PUs was likewise easily the highest, although he was only twelfth out of the 34 practices for the total number of items per 1000 PUs. Thus, Shipman prescribed high cost drugs, but not a particularly high number of drugs. Shipman's high prescribing patterns are explained by high prescribing in particular therapeutic areas. Table A.2 compares Shipman's prescribing costs with all other practices in Thameside over the period January 1995 to October 1998 for antihypertensive, bronchodilators, lipid regulating drugs and antiplatelet drugs (BNF therapeutic categories).

Shipman's cost per 1000 PUs for antiplatelet drugs is below average, but much above average for lipid regulating drugs and antihypertensives. It is also relatively high for bronchodilators.

Tables A.3, A.4 and A.5 compare Shipman's prescribing for lipid regulating, antiplatelet and antihypertensive drugs respectively for each month from January 1995 to October 1998 with all other GPs in Thameside. As far as lipid regulating drugs and antihypertensives are concerned, Shipman prescribed a higher number of items per 1000 patients earlier than his local colleagues. However, as far as antiplatelet drugs are concerned, he lagged behind his colleagues in Thameside. They almost doubled the number of items per 1000 PUs from 3.6 to 6.8, but his own rate increased only from 2.7 to 3.9 over the same period. Table A.3 shows that he was the second lowest prescriber of antiplatelet drugs among Tameside practices.

Table A.1. Summary of PPA PACT Standard Report, quarter ending September 1998, for Harold Shipman. Total list size was then 3,092, with 350 aged 65 or above, and 34 temporary residents. The number of PUs for the practice was 3,792. HS = Harold Shipman, HA=Health Authority.

| Level of suspicion | Cost (£) by BNF Group | | Number of items | | Average cost (£) | |
|---|---|---|---|---|---|---|
| | HS | HA | HS | HA | HS | HA |
| Gastro Intestinal | 10591 | 9209 | 738 | 721 | 14.35 | 12.77 |
| Cardiovascular | 41261 | 15470 | 1723 | 1885 | 23.95 | 8.21 |
| Respiratory | 21674 | 9358 | 838 | 868 | 25.86 | 10.78 |
| Central Nervous System | 17409 | 11358 | 1828 | 1787 | 9.52 | 6.36 |
| Infections | 4571 | 2859 | 743 | 654 | 6.15 | 4.37 |
| Endocrine system | 8663 | 5778 | 545 | 541 | 15.90 | 10.68 |
| All other | 19461 | 17587 | 2019 | 2208 | 9.64 | 7.97 |

Table A.2. Total prescribing costs for all practices in Thameside for the period of January 1995–October 1998.

| Practice | Total actual cost (£) | Total items | Total % generic items | Total cost per item (£) | Total items/ 1000 PUs | Total cost/ 1000 PUs (£) |
|---|---|---|---|---|---|---|
| 1 | 3215134 | 386864 | 72.7 | 8.31 | 10032 | 83380 |
| 2 | 3823675 | 513925 | 62.2 | 7.44 | 9889 | 73580 |
| 3 | 1899931 | 287474 | 56.1 | 6.61 | 8905 | 58857 |
| 4 | 1354764 | 239028 | 59.4 | 6.67 | 14753 | 83622 |
| 5 | 2915330 | 363922 | 63.1 | 8.01 | 9846 | 78878 |
| 6 | 3937174 | 623849 | 60.7 | 6.31 | 11939 | 75349 |
| 7 | 3833607 | 480986 | 57.3 | 7.97 | 10755 | 85724 |
| 8 | 2155097 | 327438 | 70.4 | 6.58 | 13645 | 89810 |
| 9 | 2713354 | 347947 | 68.6 | 7.80 | 9746 | 76004 |
| 10 | 2676151 | 426794 | 60.2 | 6.27 | 16728 | 104893 |
| 11 | 2067632 | 369780 | 64.9 | 5.59 | 10192 | 56992 |
| 12 | 3621429 | 448381 | 67.9 | 8.08 | 8301 | 67049 |
| 13 | 3337306 | 405349 | 67.7 | 8.23 | 8445 | 69534 |
| 14 | 1509655 | 193528 | 66.0 | 7.80 | 8322 | 64923 |
| 15 | 1806397 | 245945 | 63.5 | 7.34 | 9555 | 70181 |
| 16 | 2725376 | 308186 | 63.8 | 8.84 | 8883 | 78559 |
| 17 | 788255 | 98685 | 58.4 | 7.99 | 10748 | 85857 |
| 18 | 707185 | 98401 | 71.3 | 7.19 | 10160 | 73018 |
| 19 | 1451803 | 211986 | 48.8 | 6.85 | 12033 | 82409 |
| 20 | 1486042 | 202451 | 71.4 | 7.34 | 8980 | 65917 |
| 21 | 1203596 | 157182 | 70.9 | 7.66 | 10005 | 76618 |
| 22 | 1381595 | 211648 | 64.8 | 6.53 | 11416 | 74527 |
| 23 | 1392917 | 156042 | 70.2 | 8.93 | 9063 | 80903 |
| 24 | 3136726 | 449118 | 62.7 | 6.98 | 12677 | 88543 |
| 25 | 1724324 | 256584 | 71.1 | 6.72 | 12762 | 85765 |
| 26 | 928584 | 107165 | 66.4 | 8.66 | 8405 | 72830 |
| 27 | 728508 | 85396 | 61.3 | 8.53 | 8996 | 76749 |
| 28 | 881523 | 133489 | 59.9 | 6.60 | 10056 | 66409 |
| 29 | 634790 | 88246 | 73.0 | 7.19 | 12543 | 90233 |
| 30 | 395302 | 45319 | 66.9 | 8.72 | 6618 | 57733 |
| 31 | 681402 | 119706 | 56.8 | 5.69 | 11180 | 63640 |
| 32 | 549549 | 75142 | 66.9 | 7.31 | 10518 | 76924 |
| 33 | 627955 | 116241 | 61.9 | 5.4 | 13150 | 71043 |
| Shipman | 1485325 | 127795 | 71.0 | 11.62 | 10729 | 124701 |

**Table A.3. Costs of prescribing, January 1995–October 1998, for practices in Thameside (antihypertensive, bronchodilators, lipid regulating drugs, antiplatelet drugs).**

| Practice | Antihypertensives (2.5) | | Bronchodilators | | Lipid regulating drugs | | Antiplatelet drugs | |
|---|---|---|---|---|---|---|---|---|
| | Items/ 1000 PUs | Cost/ 1000 PUs (£) | Items/ 1000 PUs | Cost/ 1000 (£) | Items/ 1000 PUs | Cost/ 1000 PUs (£) | Items/ 1000 PUs | Cost/ 1000 (£) |
| 1 | 284 | 4874.58 | .55 | 5204.35 | 82 | 2349.76 | 185 | 181.97 |
| 2 | 227 | 4552.49 | .48 | 3775.17 | 78 | 1983.43 | 224 | 162.95 |
| 3 | 174 | 2060.84 | .45 | 2575.07 | 49 | 1443.18 | 177 | 165.14 |
| 4 | 215 | 4776.36 | .74 | 4053.42 | 207 | 3532.03 | 271 | 221.71 |
| 5 | 196 | 4860.63 | .50 | 3387.54 | 119 | 3249.60 | 230 | 187.32 |
| 6 | 196 | 6544.00 | .45 | 2812.63 | 119 | 2681.35 | 269 | 154.35 |
| 7 | 200 | 6248.17 | .50 | 3851.08 | 181 | 3810.01 | 273 | 217.35 |
| 8 | 353 | 4400.46 | .68 | 4589.47 | 131 | 2612.79 | 258 | 177.26 |
| 9 | 279 | 4572.98 | .52 | 4134.58 | 105 | 2654.64 | 266 | 101.33 |
| 10 | 498 | 6946.78 | 1.14 | 9048.97 | 152 | 3397.17 | 402 | 299.93 |
| 11 | 207 | 2780.38 | .51 | 3717.43 | 40 | 899.73 | 214 | 93.22 |
| 12 | 212 | 3983.42 | .42 | 3866.11 | 110 | 2974.08 | 207 | 193.44 |
| 13 | 198 | 5779.23 | .49 | 4454.58 | 136 | 3545.66 | 186 | 129.87 |
| 14 | 189 | 4511.16 | .46 | 3077.66 | 69 | 1944.97 | 185 | 132.91 |
| 15 | 145 | 4804.93 | .45 | 2382.11 | 87 | 2276.13 | 252 | 178.44 |
| 16 | 206 | 5742.49 | .44 | 4380.33 | 111 | 3041.44 | 203 | 204.98 |
| 17 | 203 | 7526.35 | .43 | 3600.26 | 107 | 4527.05 | 172 | 129.63 |
| 18 | 314 | 4027.25 | .47 | 3309.69 | 111 | 2150.44 | 320 | 194.42 |
| 19 | 152 | 4280.21 | .54 | 4481.86 | 91 | 2114.18 | 268 | 215.30 |
| 20 | 168 | 6604.83 | .40 | 2509.29 | 56 | 1944.14 | 138 | 180.70 |
| 21 | 225 | 5321.18 | .60 | 4246.73 | 68 | 1868.20 | 227 | 192.98 |
| 22 | 254 | 5575.93 | .56 | 3472.87 | 162 | 3431.20 | 259 | 153.56 |
| 23 | 209 | 5657.56 | .46 | 4571.51 | 92 | 3547.41 | 156 | 107.94 |
| 24 | 170 | 5069.18 | .47 | 3769.74 | 132 | 2545.63 | 238 | 118.74 |
| 25 | 235 | 4704.69 | .53 | 4248.82 | 100 | 2652.06 | 240 | 106.86 |
| Shipman | 241 | 20,227.34 | .50 | 7747.80 | 161 | 8851.49 | 129 | 119.89 |
| 26 | 159 | 3933.05 | .32 | 2365.58 | 162 | 4370.80 | 143 | 199.00 |
| 27 | 145 | 3520.13 | .29 | 2614.95 | 14 | 747.54 | 66 | 61.79 |
| 28 | 153 | 6184.01 | .47 | 3478.04 | 77 | 1848.88 | 155 | 147.17 |
| 29 | 240 | 9832.79 | .56 | 3856.68 | 196 | 4085.06 | 383 | 235.76 |
| 30 | 99 | 4057.03 | .26 | 3724.82 | 46 | 1827.26 | 154 | 497.35 |
| 31 | 197 | 4136.15 | .64 | 3367.39 | 111 | 2484.19 | 212 | 178.92 |
| 32 | 231 | 4477.18 | .52 | 4168.62 | 166 | 3862.26 | 211 | 117.09 |
| 33 | 217 | 4367.33 | .55 | 3511.91 | 113 | 2744.31 | 376 | 142.45 |

| Table A.4. Lipid-regulating drugs (BNF section 2.12). | | | | |
|---|---|---|---|---|
| | Harold Shipman | | Tameside GPs | |
| month | Total items | Items/ 1000 patients | Total items | Items/ 1000 patients |
| Jan–95 | 33 | 10.6 | 1246 | 5.7 |
| Feb–95 | 27 | 8.7 | 1241 | 5.7 |
| Mar–95 | 41 | 13.2 | 1485 | 6.8 |
| Apr–95 | 30 | 9.64 | 1301 | 6 |
| May–95 | 40 | 12.85 | 1473 | 6.79 |
| Jun–95 | 30 | 9.64 | 1488 | 6.86 |
| Jul–95 | 42 | 13.5 | 1476 | 6.81 |
| Aug–95 | 37 | 11.89 | 1507 | 6.95 |
| Sep–95 | 29 | 9.32 | 1500 | 6.92 |
| Oct–95 | 40 | 13.09 | 1518 | 7.05 |
| Nov–95 | 39 | 12.77 | 1610 | 7.48 |
| Dec–95 | 41 | 13.42 | 1582 | 7.35 |
| Jan–96 | 48 | 15.71 | 1643 | 7.59 |
| Feb–96 | 41 | 13.42 | 1653 | 7.64 |
| Mar–96 | 44 | 14.4 | 1709 | 7.89 |
| Apr–96 | 44 | 14.42 | 1720 | 7.98 |
| May–96 | 42 | 13.76 | 1816 | 8.43 |
| Jun–96 | 45 | 14.74 | 1702 | 7.9 |
| Jul–96 | 39 | 12.68 | 1891 | 8.78 |
| Aug–96 | 38 | 12.35 | 1919 | 8.91 |
| Sep–96 | 44 | 14.3 | 1754 | 8.15 |
| Oct–96 | 38 | 12.45 | 2032 | 9.43 |
| Nov–96 | 37 | 12.12 | 1931 | 8.96 |
| Dec–96 | 40 | 13.1 | 2055 | 9.54 |
| Jan–97 | 36 | 11.62 | 2029 | 9.42 |
| Feb–97 | 37 | 11.95 | 1899 | 8.82 |
| Mar–97 | 44 | 14.21 | 1941 | 9.01 |
| Apr–97 | 38 | 12.45 | 2234 | 10.43 |
| May–97 | 47 | 15.39 | 2228 | 10.4 |
| Jun–97 | 38 | 12.45 | 2109 | 9.85 |
| Jul–97 | 45 | 14.71 | 2365 | 11.03 |
| Aug–97 | 35 | 11.44 | 2277 | 10.62 |
| Sep–97 | 52 | 17 | 2329 | 10.86 |
| Oct–97 | 46 | 15.12 | 2463 | 11.48 |
| Nov–97 | 43 | 14.14 | 2378 | 11.08 |
| Dec–97 | 51 | 16.77 | 2602 | 12.13 |
| Jan–98 | 50 | 16.48 | 2488 | 11.62 |
| Feb–98 | 41 | 13.51 | 2439 | 11.39 |
| Mar–98 | 62 | 20.44 | 2698 | 12.6 |
| Apr–98 | 43 | 14.17 | 2737 | 12.83 |
| May–98 | 46 | 15.16 | 2689 | 12.61 |
| Jun–98 | 44 | 14.5 | 2761 | 12.95 |
| Jul–98 | 57 | 18.43 | 3053 | 14.29 |
| Aug–98 | 51 | 16.49 | 2818 | 13.19 |
| Sep–98 | 40 | 12.94 | 3031 | 14.19 |
| Oct–98 | 48 | 15.95 | 3143 | 14.72 |

**Table A.5. Prescribing of antiplatelet drugs (BNF section 2.9) by Harold Shipman and Tameside GPs (excluding Shipman), January 1995–October 1998, indicating total items prescribed per month and items per 1000 PUs.**

| month | Tameside GPs | | Harold Shipman | |
|---|---|---|---|---|
| | Total items | Items/ 1000 PUs | Total items | Items/ 1000 PUs |
| Jan–95 | 3177 | 3.6 | 32 | 2.7 |
| Feb–95 | 2990 | 3.4 | 31 | 2.6 |
| Mar–95 | 3570 | 4.0 | 30 | 2.5 |
| Apr–95 | 3198 | 3.6 | 22 | 1.8 |
| May–95 | 3440 | 3.9 | 29 | 2.4 |
| Jun–95 | 3606 | 4.1 | 30 | 2.5 |
| Jul–95 | 3547 | 4.0 | 25 | 2.1 |
| Aug–95 | 3690 | 4.2 | 24 | 2.0 |
| Sep–95 | 3622 | 4.1 | 31 | 2.6 |
| Oct–95 | 3680 | 4.2 | 25 | 2.1 |
| Nov–95 | 3887 | 4.4 | 26 | 2.2 |
| Dec–95 | 3791 | 4.3 | 26 | 2.2 |
| Jan–96 | 3909 | 4.4 | 35 | 2.9 |
| Feb–96 | 3878 | 4.4 | 18 | 1.5 |
| Mar–96 | 3946 | 4.5 | 29 | 2.4 |
| Apr–96 | 4119 | 4.7 | 31 | 2.6 |
| May–96 | 4387 | 5.0 | 30 | 2.5 |
| Jun–96 | 3976 | 4.5 | 31 | 2.6 |
| Jul–96 | 4530 | 5.1 | 46 | 3.8 |
| Aug–96 | 4361 | 4.9 | 29 | 2.4 |
| Sep–96 | 4208 | 4.8 | 32 | 2.7 |
| Oct–96 | 4581 | 5.2 | 40 | 3.3 |
| Nov–96 | 4380 | 4.9 | 36 | 3.0 |
| Dec–96 | 4481 | 5.1 | 31 | 2.6 |
| Jan–97 | 4624 | 5.2 | 42 | 3.5 |
| Feb–97 | 4197 | 4.7 | 31 | 2.6 |
| Mar–97 | 4293 | 4.8 | 35 | 2.9 |
| Apr–97 | 4728 | 5.3 | 29 | 2.4 |
| May–97 | 4686 | 5.3 | 38 | 3.1 |
| Jun–97 | 4593 | 5.2 | 31 | 2.6 |
| Jul–97 | 4999 | 5.7 | 37 | 3.1 |
| Aug–97 | 4700 | 5.3 | 34 | 2.8 |
| Sep–97 | 4887 | 5.5 | 33 | 2.8 |
| Oct–97 | 5154 | 5.8 | 37 | 3.1 |
| Nov–97 | 4819 | 5.5 | 30 | 2.5 |
| Dec–97 | 5388 | 6.1 | 38 | 3.2 |
| Jan–98 | 5054 | 5.7 | 34 | 2.8 |
| Feb–98 | 4673 | 5.3 | 33 | 2.7 |
| Mar–98 | 5309 | 6.0 | 36 | 3.0 |
| Apr–98 | 5422 | 6.1 | 43 | 3.6 |
| May–98 | 5208 | 5.9 | 34 | 2.8 |
| Jun–98 | 5307 | 6.0 | 50 | 4.2 |
| Jul–98 | 5876 | 6.6 | 44 | 3.6 |
| Aug–98 | 5388 | 6.1 | 33 | 2.7 |
| Sep–98 | 5831 | 6.6 | 45 | 3.7 |
| Oct–98 | 6007 | 6.8 | 46 | 3.9 |

Table A.6. Prescribing of antihypertensives (BNF section 2.5) by Harold Shipman and Tameside GPs (excluding Shipman), January 1995–October 1998, indicating total items prescribed per month and items per 1000 PUs.

| month | Tameside GPs | | Harold Shipman | |
|---|---|---|---|---|
| | Total items | Items/ 1000 PUs | Total items | Items/ 1000 PUs |
| Jan–95 | 5302 | 6.0 | 134 | 11.1 |
| Feb–95 | 5009 | 5.7 | 105 | 8.7 |
| Mar–95 | 5921 | 6.7 | 137 | 11.3 |
| Apr–95 | 5423 | 6.1 | 118 | 9.8 |
| May–95 | 5846 | 6.6 | 152 | 12.6 |
| Jun–95 | 5956 | 6.7 | 144 | 11.9 |
| Jul–95 | 5774 | 6.5 | 140 | 11.6 |
| Aug–95 | 5970 | 6.7 | 123 | 10.2 |
| Sep–95 | 5709 | 6.4 | 136 | 11.2 |
| Oct–95 | 5890 | 6.6 | 162 | 13.4 |
| Nov–95 | 6137 | 6.9 | 148 | 12.2 |
| Dec–95 | 6078 | 6.9 | 152 | 12.6 |
| Jan–96 | 6088 | 6.9 | 170 | 14.0 |
| Feb–96 | 6129 | 6.9 | 148 | 12.2 |
| Mar–96 | 6185 | 7.0 | 181 | 15.0 |
| Apr–96 | 6289 | 7.1 | 159 | 13.1 |
| May–96 | 6706 | 7.6 | 170 | 14.0 |
| Jun–96 | 5955 | 6.7 | 131 | 10.8 |
| Jul–96 | 6669 | 7.5 | 169 | 14.0 |
| Aug–96 | 6586 | 7.4 | 161 | 13.3 |
| Sep–96 | 6132 | 6.9 | 145 | 12.0 |
| Oct–96 | 6855 | 7.7 | 171 | 14.1 |
| Nov–96 | 6616 | 7.5 | 164 | 13.6 |
| Dec–96 | 6746 | 7.6 | 149 | 12.3 |
| Jan–97 | 6781 | 7.7 | 151 | 12.5 |
| Feb–97 | 6196 | 7.0 | 132 | 10.9 |
| Mar–97 | 6345 | 7.2 | 164 | 13.6 |
| Apr–97 | 7040 | 8.0 | 168 | 13.9 |
| May–97 | 7146 | 8.1 | 172 | 14.2 |
| Jun–97 | 6679 | 7.6 | 171 | 14.2 |
| Jul–97 | 7258 | 8.2 | 159 | 13.2 |
| Aug–97 | 6711 | 7.6 | 155 | 12.9 |
| Sep–97 | 7003 | 7.9 | 162 | 13.5 |
| Oct–97 | 7344 | 8.3 | 177 | 14.8 |
| Nov–97 | 6919 | 7.8 | 155 | 12.9 |
| Dec–97 | 7567 | 8.6 | 177 | 14.8 |
| Jan–98 | 7235 | 8.2 | 172 | 14.3 |
| Feb–98 | 6554 | 7.4 | 160 | 13.3 |
| Mar–98 | 7597 | 8.6 | 181 | 15.0 |
| Apr–98 | 7547 | 8.5 | 177 | 14.7 |
| May–98 | 7441 | 8.4 | 170 | 14.1 |
| Jun–98 | 7558 | 8.6 | 165 | 13.7 |
| Jul–98 | 8187 | 9.3 | 193 | 15.9 |
| Aug–98 | 7393 | 8.4 | 179 | 14.8 |
| Sep–98 | 7936 | 9.0 | 186 | 15.4 |
| Oct–98 | 8028 | 9.1 | 167 | 14.0 |

Table A.7. Prescribing of inhaled corticosteroids (BNF section 3.2) by Harold Shipman and Tameside GPs (excluding Shipman), January 1995–October 1998, indicating total items prescribed per month and items per 1000 PUs.

| month | Tameside GPs | | Harold Shipman | |
|---|---|---|---|---|
| | Total items | Items/ 1000 PUs | Total items | Items/ 1000 PUs |
| Jan–95 | 3827 | 4.3 | 64 | 5.3 |
| Feb–95 | 3440 | 3.9 | 47 | 3.9 |
| Mar–95 | 4086 | 4.6 | 66 | 5.5 |
| Apr–95 | 3499 | 3.9 | 64 | 5.3 |
| May–95 | 4026 | 4.5 | 64 | 5.3 |
| Jun–95 | 4157 | 4.7 | 61 | 5.0 |
| Jul–95 | 3931 | 4.4 | 71 | 5.9 |
| Aug–95 | 3890 | 4.4 | 49 | 4.0 |
| Sep–95 | 3853 | 4.3 | 60 | 5.0 |
| Oct–95 | 3854 | 4.3 | 73 | 6.0 |
| Nov–95 | 4186 | 4.7 | 78 | 6.4 |
| Dec–95 | 4154 | 4.7 | 62 | 5.1 |
| Jan–96 | 4071 | 4.6 | 70 | 5.8 |
| Feb–96 | 3973 | 4.4 | 65 | 5.4 |
| Mar–96 | 4009 | 4.5 | 62 | 5.1 |
| Apr–96 | 3915 | 4.4 | 62 | 5.1 |
| May–96 | 4233 | 4.8 | 65 | 5.4 |
| Jun–96 | 3888 | 4.4 | 59 | 4.9 |
| Jul–96 | 4464 | 5.0 | 57 | 4.7 |
| Aug–96 | 3961 | 4.5 | 53 | 4.4 |
| Sep–96 | 3985 | 4.5 | 58 | 4.8 |
| Oct–96 | 4361 | 4.9 | 52 | 4.3 |
| Nov–96 | 4403 | 5.0 | 49 | 4.0 |
| Dec–96 | 4508 | 5.2 | 62 | 5.1 |
| Jan–97 | 4513 | 5.1 | 56 | 4.6 |
| Feb–97 | 4022 | 4.5 | 62 | 5.1 |
| Mar–97 | 4082 | 4.6 | 48 | 4.0 |
| Apr–97 | 4429 | 5.0 | 56 | 4.6 |
| May–97 | 4489 | 5.1 | 66 | 5.5 |
| Jun–97 | 4223 | 4.8 | 53 | 4.4 |
| Jul–97 | 4534 | 5.1 | 64 | 5.3 |
| Aug–97 | 4117 | 4.7 | 66 | 5.5 |
| Sep–97 | 4568 | 5.2 | 52 | 4.3 |
| Oct–97 | 4809 | 5.4 | 76 | 6.3 |
| Nov–97 | 4475 | 5.1 | 61 | 5.1 |
| Dec–97 | 5073 | 5.7 | 77 | 6.4 |
| Jan–98 | 4607 | 5.2 | 63 | 5.2 |
| Feb–98 | 4336 | 4.9 | 64 | 5.3 |
| Mar–98 | 4645 | 5.3 | 58 | 4.8 |
| Apr–98 | 4524 | 5.1 | 72 | 6.0 |
| May–98 | 4554 | 5.2 | 67 | 5.6 |
| Jun–98 | 4616 | 5.2 | 65 | 5.4 |
| Jul–98 | 4903 | 5.5 | 77 | 6.4 |
| Aug–98 | 4193 | 4.7 | 55 | 4.5 |
| Sep–98 | 4768 | 5.4 | 69 | 5.7 |
| Oct–98 | 4874 | 5.5 | 66 | 5.5 |

| Table A.8. Hypnotics and anxiolytics (BNF section 4.1). Number of items prescribed by Shipman and cost per month and cost per item, January 1995–October 1998. | | | |
|---|---|---|---|
| month | cost | items | cost/item |
| Jan–95 | 425.35 | 115 | 3.7 |
| Feb–95 | 290.71 | 102 | 2.85 |
| Mar–95 | 449.01 | 121 | 3.71 |
| Apr–95 | 331.36 | 108 | 3.07 |
| May–95 | 361.5 | 127 | 2.85 |
| Jun–95 | 317.12 | 115 | 2.76 |
| Jul–95 | 322.74 | 108 | 2.99 |
| Aug–95 | 328.4 | 116 | 2.83 |
| Sep–95 | 430.99 | 120 | 3.59 |
| Oct–95 | 283.9 | 110 | 2.58 |
| Nov–95 | 331.42 | 117 | 2.83 |
| Dec–95 | 394.17 | 126 | 3.13 |
| Jan–96 | 363.93 | 125 | 2.91 |
| Feb–96 | 352.12 | 122 | 2.89 |
| Mar–96 | 300.87 | 100 | 3.01 |
| Apr–96 | 352.18 | 122 | 2.89 |
| May–96 | 369.78 | 125 | 2.96 |
| Jun–96 | 391.69 | 124 | 3.16 |
| Jul–96 | 435.05 | 133 | 3.27 |
| Aug–96 | 311.7 | 128 | 2.44 |
| Sep–96 | 395.19 | 119 | 3.32 |
| Oct–96 | 417.59 | 131 | 3.19 |
| Nov–96 | 321.15 | 124 | 2.59 |
| Dec–96 | 345.55 | 121 | 2.86 |
| Jan–97 | 414.5 | 122 | 3.4 |
| Feb–97 | 288.75 | 112 | 2.58 |
| Mar–97 | 296.22 | 104 | 2.85 |
| Apr–97 | 381.92 | 130 | 2.94 |
| May–97 | 304.39 | 94 | 3.24 |
| Jun–97 | 305.09 | 105 | 2.91 |
| Jul–97 | 332.87 | 109 | 3.05 |
| Aug–97 | 269.69 | 112 | 2.41 |
| Sep–97 | 279.12 | 108 | 2.58 |
| Oct–97 | 332.88 | 113 | 2.95 |
| Nov–97 | 265.32 | 113 | 2.35 |
| Dec–97 | 326.8 | 114 | 2.87 |
| Jan–98 | 317.13 | 118 | 2.69 |
| Feb–98 | 315.25 | 114 | 2.77 |
| Mar–98 | 199.78 | 95 | 2.1 |
| Apr–98 | 243.62 | 119 | 2.05 |
| May–98 | 160.97 | 103 | 1.56 |
| Jun–98 | 269.5 | 122 | 2.21 |
| Jul–98 | 224.44 | 132 | 1.7 |
| Aug–98 | 240.47 | 132 | 1.82 |
| Sep–98 | 216.96 | 125 | 1.74 |
| Oct–98 | 133.48 | 89 | 1.5 |

Table A.6 shows the same information for prescribing of inhaled corticosteroids, and no differences are evident between Shipman's prescribing habits and other Thameside GPs.

Table A.7 and A.8 give the number of items and cost per 1000 PUs for practices in Hyde for the period January 1995 to October 1998 for drugs used in substance dependence, and analgesics, treatment of obesity, antidepressants, antipsychotics, hypnotics and anxiolytics. Shipman's prescribing is the most expensive for three of these categories: drugs used in substance dependence, antidepressants, hypnotics and anxiolytics.

Table A.9 shows the number of prescriptions for drugs in the six categories issued by Shipman between January 1995 and October 1998 by month. The table suggests a trend towards increase prescribing of antidepressants, no particular pattern for analgesics, a trend to towards increased use of antipsychotics, no general trend for hypnotics and anxiolytics, and also no clear trend for drugs for substance dependence.

In summary, therefore Shipman was a particularly high cost prescriber. This was particularly marked in certain therapeutic areas, for example antihypertensive, lipid regulating drugs, and antidepressants. This pattern suggest that he prescribed relatively new and more expensive medications more readily than most general practitioners, although was slower than other local general practitioners to increase the rate of prescribing of antiplatelet drugs.

**Table A.9.**

| Practice | Drugs used in substance dependence (4.10) | | Analgesics (4.7) | | Treatment of obesity (4.5) | |
|---|---|---|---|---|---|---|
| | Items/ 1000 PUs | Cost/ 1000 PUs (£) | Items/ 1000 PUs | Cost/ 1000 PUs (£) | Items/ 1000 PUs | Cost/ 1000 PUs (£) |
| 1 | 23.8 | 165.53 | 0.83 | 4586.95 | 11.1 | 40.03 |
| 9 | 18.6 | 99.29 | 0.79 | 4201.42 | 0.3 | 1.61 |
| 13 | 46.7 | 205.90 | 0.77 | 2988.81 | 0.4 | 3.35 |
| Shipman | 75.6 | 356.80 | 1.03 | 4678.35 | 2.2 | 13.30 |

**Table A.10.**

| Practice | Antidepressants (4.3) | | Antipsychotics (4.2) | | Hypnotics & anxiolytics (4.1) | |
|---|---|---|---|---|---|---|
| | Items/ 1000 PUs | Cost/ 1000 PUs (£) | Items/ 1000 PUs | Cost/ 1000 PUs (£) | Items/ 1000 PUs | Cost/ 1000 PUs (£) |
| 1 | 316 | 3827.11 | 79 | 880.28 | 454 | 596.49 |
| 9 | 297 | 4526.74 | 108 | 576.44 | 355 | 364.26 |
| 13 | 243 | 2926.02 | 74 | 450.49 | 385 | 581.19 |
| Shipman | 295 | 6464.84 | 72 | 326.01 | 449 | 1237.73 |

| Table A.11. Numbered items prescribed by Shipman each month 1995–98, for selected drug categories. | | | | | |
|---|---|---|---|---|---|
| month | Anti-depressants | Analgesics | Anti-psychotics | Hypnotics & anxiolytics | Substance dependence |
| Jan–95 | 62 | 264 | 12 | 115 | 9 |
| Feb–95 | 66 | 315 | 9 | 102 | 8 |
| Mar–95 | 77 | 305 | 17 | 121 | 13 |
| Apr–95 | 64 | 215 | 14 | 108 | 14 |
| May–95 | 69 | 249 | 12 | 127 | 16 |
| Jun–95 | 58 | 213 | 14 | 115 | 24 |
| Jul–95 | 51 | 236 | 17 | 108 | 20 |
| Aug–95 | 44 | 193 | 8 | 116 | 17 |
| Sep–95 | 71 | 237 | 11 | 120 | 20 |
| Oct–95 | 61 | 247 | 10 | 110 | 20 |
| Nov–95 | 65 | 336 | 9 | 117 | 21 |
| Dec–95 | 73 | 323 | 12 | 126 | 21 |
| Jan–96 | 63 | 283 | 10 | 125 | 23 |
| Feb–96 | 76 | 256 | 14 | 122 | 21 |
| Mar–96 | 65 | 264 | 15 | 100 | 23 |
| Apr–96 | 69 | 267 | 13 | 122 | 23 |
| May–96 | 68 | 302 | 18 | 125 | 25 |
| Jun–96 | 68 | 226 | 15 | 124 | 21 |
| Jul–96 | 83 | 286 | 11 | 133 | 19 |
| Aug–96 | 68 | 191 | 19 | 128 | 24 |
| Sep–96 | 67 | 227 | 16 | 119 | 16 |
| Oct–96 | 72 | 284 | 16 | 131 | 22 |
| Nov–96 | 75 | 277 | 15 | 124 | 28 |
| Dec–96 | 76 | 393 | 15 | 121 | 26 |
| Jan–97 | 74 | 304 | 11 | 122 | 23 |
| Feb–97 | 72 | 285 | 18 | 112 | 20 |
| Mar–97 | 74 | 236 | 18 | 104 | 19 |
| Apr–97 | 83 | 276 | 19 | 130 | 18 |
| May–97 | 81 | 287 | 25 | 94 | 20 |
| Jun–97 | 66 | 250 | 27 | 105 | 17 |
| Jul–97 | 83 | 258 | 28 | 109 | 17 |
| Aug–97 | 87 | 205 | 26 | 112 | 17 |
| Sep–97 | 83 | 251 | 22 | 108 | 22 |
| Oct–97 | 93 | 314 | 26 | 113 | 20 |
| Nov–97 | 87 | 274 | 22 | 113 | 22 |
| Dec–97 | 89 | 334 | 33 | 114 | 24 |
| Jan–98 | 82 | 284 | 23 | 118 | 22 |
| Feb–98 | 76 | 286 | 22 | 114 | 23 |
| Mar–98 | 81 | 289 | 33 | 95 | 17 |
| Apr–98 | 85 | 272 | 26 | 119 | 17 |
| May–98 | 84 | 244 | 27 | 103 | 18 |
| Jun–98 | 98 | 274 | 34 | 122 | 19 |
| Jul–98 | 113 | 268 | 31 | 132 | 19 |
| Aug–98 | 112 | 241 | 22 | 132 | 15 |
| Sep–98 | 107 | 223 | 27 | 125 | 18 |
| Oct–98 | 96 | 217 | 18 | 89 | 19 |

# Appendix 4. Audits reported to West Pennine Primary Care Clinical Audit Group

From 1991, general practitioners were encouraged to take part in clinical audit, and local groups were created to support audit – medical audit advisory groups (MAAGs). Tameside MAAG was Shipman's local group. This MAAG encouraged practitioners to report their audits to them, and also instituted a programme of visits to practices to assess their audit activities. In later years, visits were replaced by a questionnaire on audit activity completed by the practice. A summary of the audits reported to the MAAG by Shipman's practice is included below.

## Level of activity

Tameside MAAG's report for 1993/94 indicates that audits had been undertaken by the practice. The practice was visited in February 1993, when audit activity was reported to have led to change in care. A computer system was to be installed in the next few months, and the premises were being improved to provide new facilities – a staff room, computer room and midwive's consulting room. The report concludes: "An enthusiastic practice where we were warmly received and audit is clearly an integral part of the work."

A second visit took place on in February 1994. The report indicates that audits were being undertaken concerned with a variety of topics including benzodiazepine prescribing, chronic disease management, congestive cardiac failure and patient deaths. Other audits were planned, and the practice was involved in a total quality management project sponsored by the local Family Health Services Authority (FHSA). The practice was judged to be highly motivated – "This practice displays an enthusiasm for audit and quality deliverance of care. Audit has become a meaningful integrated part of general practice."

A self-complete questionnaire was used in 1994/5 to assess practice audit activity. Dr Shipman refers to the epilepsy, 16 year olds and repeat appointment projects again. He had only taken part in one of the four audits organised by the MAAG – benzodiazepine use.

The audit activity questionnaire for 1995/6 indicated that 11 audits had been taking place, addressing clinical topics that included asthma in adults, diabetes, migraine and benign prostatic hypertrophy. The responses to the questionnaire generally show a positive attitude towards audit, and appears to have been completed by a practice nurse.

A positive note is also found in the 1996/7 audit activity questionnaire. The respondent reported that audits had led to improvements in the quality of care provided, administrative procedures, teamwork, communication and awareness of what was happening in the practice. Several audits had been undertaken, and the practice was willing to share the findings with other practices. Of the five audits organised by the audit group, the practice had only taken part in that for diabetes. When asked about activities that the audit group could undertake, the respondent suggested that practice visits should be organised every two years.

A practice audit activity questionnaire was also completed for 1997/8. Several guidelines were reported as being used in the practice, but the questionnaire does not include detailed information about audits.

A further visit by the audit group to the practice was made in January 1998. Dr Shipman and the practice nurse were present at the visit. Seven audits were reviewed. The report comments: 'Great to see a single-handed enthusiastic GP with a rolling programme of audit. Practice Nurse also very enthusiastic and takes part in audit. We think it would be very useful for you to have an Audit Assistant and hope you follow this up. Keep up the good work!'.

## Audit of care of patients with epilepsy

The date of the audit is uncertain, but is likely to be early – 1992/3. The report held by the Tameside MAAG is a simple first data collection, typical of practice audits of that time. The audit had no criteria or standards.

The practice disease register is reported as complete. 29 patients with epilepsy were identified (0.9% of the practice list). Patients were invited to attend for review. Sixteen patients were given advice on driving, three had changes to their medication and one received advice about compliance. It is claimed that no patient had had "any more fits since they were seen".

In 1994, patients with epilepsy were sent letters to offer them a review, to be undertaken according to a practice protocol. There were 33 patients on this occasion.

## High vaginal swabs

A small project was undertaken in 1992/3. A comparison was made between preliminary clinical and eventual microbiological diagnoses. The conclusion was that high vaginal swabs for culture was of little value.

## Audit of district nurses in the surgery

This project was undertaken in 1992/3. Shipman did not have a district nurse for patients to consult on the practice premises. He had open access consultation sessions and dealt with patients who might otherwise consult a district nurse. He concluded from his findings that a district nurse working in the practice was not required.

## Repeat appointments

In 1994 Dr Shipman collected information about the number of appointments that were for follow up of patients with existing problems. His data collection lasted for one month; 41% of consultations were follow ups.

## Asthma

An assessment of the symptoms of people with asthma was undertaken in 1994. The report of the audit includes summary data only and there is no description of methods. Therefore, it is not possible to draw any conclusions from the information available.

## Survey of 16 year olds

In 1993, Shipman asked Tameside MAAG whether it would award him £200 to support a survey of 16 year olds in his practice. The aims of the project were to identify health problems and provide appropriate advice. The project appears to have been completed. Twenty-three of 32 patients invited for assessment eventually attended. Many received advice about lifestyle. The investigations included cholesterol level.

## Asthma audit

Another audit of the care of people with asthma is reported on a standard form, presumably that of the local MAAG. The audit may have been a multi-practice audit organised by the audit group. Forty-four patients were included, and the findings indicate a reasonable level of care with improvement during the audit. For example, the proportion of patients with symptoms suggestive of poor disease control reduced during the audit.

## Audit of cholesterol management after myocardial infarction

In an audit dated to 1997, 25 patients aged less than 70 were identified as having had a myocardial infarction. The cholesterol levels of all these patients had been tested in the previous 18 months. Four of the six patients who had a cholesterol level above 6.0 mml/l were not receiving medication, but plans were reported for reviewing these patients.

## Patients leaving the practice

An audit reported to the audit group in November 1997 was concerned with patients who left the practice. The total number of patients leaving the practice was not given, but 37.5% of removals were due to external transfers (to another health authority), deaths accounted for 27.9%, other removals 18.3% and internal transfers (within the same health authority) 16.3%. The report announced plans to send questionnaires to internal transfers to investigate the reason for changing GP.

## New Patient Registrations

This audit was reported in July 1998. The aim was to ensure that all new patients were entered onto the practice computer and that immunisation and cervical cytology histories were recorded. It was practice policy that all new patients should be seen by the GP before being accepted onto the list. The findings confirmed that patients were being recorded on the computer, but that immunisation and cervical cytology histories were sometimes incomplete. The problem was believed to be due to the slow transfer of patient medical records from the patient's previous practice.

## Steriods and osteoporosis

This audit was reported in 1998. The practice determined that patients who received steroids for 12 months or longer should be offered osteoporosis prevention treatment. Three of the 13 patients identified were found to be receiving medication to reduce the risk of osteoporosis, and plans to review the remaining patients were described.

# Appendix 5. Reviews of the care of people with angina or diabetes registered with The Surgery, 21 Market Street, Hyde

## 1 Review of care of patients with angina

### Background

Angina is a clinical syndrome usually caused by coronary artery disease. Patients with angina are at increased risk of death from myocardial infarction, and their continuing care is largely undertaken by general practitioners. A relatively high proportion of the MCCDs issued by Shipman gave myocardial infarction or ischaemic heart disease as the cause of death and therefore a review was undertaken of the care of people with angina who were registered with the practice in Hyde.

### Methods

The review only included patients who had been registered in the practice before September 1998 and had also had angina diagnosed before that date. They would therefore have received care from Shipman.

The review was undertaken using a standard audit protocol (Khunti et al, 1995). This was selected because it would have been current up to Shipman's arrest and had been developed following review of research evidence. The protocol includes full instructions for identifying patients and collecting data. The review criteria are classified into two levels (Box A.1) – 'must do' (the minimum criteria that practices need to audit as there is firm research evidence to justify their inclusion) and 'should do' (there is some research evidence of their importance).

Data about the care provided before 7th September 1998 were collected from clinical records by the doctors working in the practice (Dr Wilson and Dr Hannan) in order to ensure patient confidentiality (GMC, 2000). They provided anonymised information on recording forms, from which the proportions whose care was in accordance with each criterion was calculated.

| Box A.1. The criteria used in the review of care of people with angina. |
|---|
| **'Must do'** |
| 1.  The records show that the diagnosis of angina is based on: (a) characteristic symptoms of angina or (b) suggestive symptoms of angina supported by positive investigations. |
| 2.  The records show that at diagnosis the blood pressure has been recorded, the patient examined for signs of anaemia, and has had a cardiac examination. |
| 3.  The records show that the patient is on daily aspirin unless contraindicated. |
| 4.  The records show that at least annually there has been an assessment of smoking habit, and advice given to smokers. |
| 5.  The records show that at diagnosis the patient's blood lipids have been checked. |
| 6.  The records show that at least annually the blood pressure has been checked and is within normal limits. |
| 7.  The records show that there is an annual assessment of symptoms. |
| **'Should do'** |
| 8.  The records show that at least annually regular physical activity has been discussed with the patient. |
| 9.  The records show that the body mass index is checked at diagnosis. |
| 10.  The records show that the patient has had a resting 12 lead ECG. |

# Findings

Table A.12 presents information about the patients with angina including their medical and surgical management. Tables A.13 and 14 present the numbers and percentages of patients whose care was in accordance with the 'must do' and 'should do' criteria respectively.

| Table A.12. Background information about the patients with angina included in the audit (CABG = coronary artery bypass graft; GTN = glyceryl trinitrate). | | |
|---|---|---|
| | number | % |
| **Gender** | | |
| Male | 13 | 50.0 |
| Female | 13 | 50.0 |
| Year of diagnosis | | |
| 1970–1979 | 2 | 7.7 |
| 1980–1989 | 10 | 38.5 |
| 1990–1998 | 14 | 53.8 |
| **Surgical treatment** | | |
| CABG | 7 | 26.9 |
| **Medical treatment** | | |
| None | 2 | 7.7 |
| GTN only | 2 | 7.7 |
| GTN plus ß blocker and/or calcium channel blocker | 15 | 57.7 |
| Other | 7 | 26.9 |

| Table A.13. The numbers and percentages of patients whose care was in accordance with the 'Must do' criteria. | | |
|---|---|---|
| **Criterion** | **number** | **%** |
| **Criterion 1** | | |
| *characteristic symptoms* | | |
| Yes | 17 | 65.4 |
| No | 3 | 11.5 |
| not known | 6 | 23.1 |
| *suggestive symptoms in those without characteristic symptoms* | | |
| Yes | 3 | 100 |
| *referred for investigations* | | |
| Yes | 16 | 61.5 |
| No | 9 | 34.6 |
| not known | 1 | 3.8 |
| | | |
| **Criterion 2** | | |
| *BP checked at diagnosis* | | |
| Yes | 9 | 34.6 |
| No | 13 | 50.0 |
| not known | 4 | 15.4 |
| *examined for anaemia at diagnosis* | | |
| Yes | 1 | 3.8 |
| No | 20 | 76.9 |
| not known | 5 | 19.2 |
| *cardiac examination at diagnosis* | | |
| Yes | 7 | 26.9 |
| No | 13 | 50.0 |
| not known | 6 | 23.1 |
| | | |
| **Criterion 3** | | |
| *On daily aspirin* | | |
| Yes | 20 | 76.9 |
| No | 6 | 23.1 |
| | | |
| **Criterion 4** | | |
| *Smoking habit checked annually* | | |
| yes, smoker, advice given | 5 | 19.2 |
| yes, non-smoker | 2 | 7.7 |
| No | 10 | 38.5 |
| not known | 9 | 34.6 |
| | | |
| **Criterion 5** | | |
| *lipids checked at diagnosis* | | |
| Yes | 4 | 15.4 |
| | | |
| **Criterion 6** | | |
| *annual BP check* | | |
| yes, result normal | 12 | 46.2 |
| yes, result above 160/90 | 6 | 23.1 |
| No | 8 | 30.8 |
| | | |
| **Criterion 7** | | |
| *annual assessment of symptoms* | | |
| Yes | 16 | 61.5 |
| No | 3 | 11.5 |
| not known | 7 | 26.9 |

**Table A.14. The numbers and percentages of patients whose care was in accordance with the 'Should do' criteria.**

| Criterion | number | % |
|---|---|---|
| **Criterion 8** | | |
| *Annual discussion of physical activity* | | |
| yes | 3 | 11.5 |
| no | 14 | 53.8 |
| not known | 9 | 34.6 |
| | | |
| **Criterion 9** | | |
| *BMI checked in past year* | | |
| yes | 8 | 30.8 |
| no | 18 | 69.2 |
| | | |
| **Criterion 10** | | |
| *12 lead ECG performed* | | |
| yes, abnormal | 6 | 23.1 |
| yes, normal | 7 | 26.9 |
| yes, result not known | 2 | 7.7 |
| no | 10 | 38.5 |
| not known | 1 | 3.8 |

## Conclusions

In evaluating the care provided by Shipman to patients with angina, several aspects of the audit should be borne in mind. The patients who were included were those who had not died or changed to another practice since Shipman's arrest. The findings relate to the care given until September 1998 and do not reflect the care provided since then. Shipman's recording habits were less than satisfactory, and some of the findings may simply be due to poor recording. Subject to these qualifications, the level of compliance with the 'must do' audit criteria is, with some exceptions, likely to be regarded as unremarkable.

In all those cases containing adequate information in the records to enable a judgement to be drawn, symptoms to support a diagnosis of angina were recorded. Furthermore, 61.5% of patients had been referred to a specialist. In contrast, the records often did not contain a record of a full assessment at the time of diagnosis (criterion two).

Relatively few published audits of the primary care of people with angina are available to provide comparative data against which to judge Shipman's performance. However, several audits have been reported relating to the prescribing of aspirin (criterion three). Forty-seven practices in Liverpool took part in a programme to increase the proportion of patients with coronary artery disease prescribed aspirin in general practice. The percentage of such patients initially receiving aspirin ranged from 15% to 75% (Wilcox et al, 1996). Information from five audits, each involving from 20 to 45 general practices and from 290 to 4602 patients, reported that the proportions of patients in each audit who were taking aspirin varied from 52% to 84% (Clinical Governance Research and Development Unit, 1999). Thus, the level of 76.9% achieved among Shipman's patients was reasonable.

The records did not indicate regular assessment of smoking habits (criterion four) or checks of serum lipids (criterion five), although blood pressure (criterion six) and symptoms (criterion seven) were more likely to be recorded as having being assessed. Levels of compliance with the 'should do' criteria tended to be low, although 58% of patients had been investigated with an ECG.

The findings therefore indicate that although several aspects of care could be improved, it would have been unlikely for them to have been regarded during the mid 1990s as indicating a distinct outlier practice in comparison with other practices.

# 2    Audit of care for people with diabetes

## Background

Approximately 2% of the population have diabetes, although it is more common in people over aged 65. The consequences for affected individuals include an increased risk of death from myocardial infarction, and complications that include renal, vascular and neurological problems. Primary health care teams have a major role in the detection and continued management of people with diabetes, and therefore a review of the care of people with diabetes at The Surgery in Hyde was undertaken.

## Method

A standard audit protocol was used (Baker et al, 1993). It was chosen because it had been used in audits by large numbers of practices, had been developed following review of relevant research evidence, and would have been current during Shipman's clinical practice. The protocol includes review criteria (Box A.2), instructions for identifying patients and collecting data, and data collection forms.

Patients were included if they were known to have diabetes and had been registered with the practice prior to September 1998. The data collection was undertaken in the practice by the practice nurse in order to ensure patient confidentiality. Information was sought about care delivered up to September 1998, and therefore the findings relate to care during Shipman's period in the practice. The resulting anonymous data were used to calculate the proportions of patients whose care was in accordance with the criteria.

| Box A.2. The criteria used in the review of care of people with diabetes. |
|---|

| | 'Must do' |
|---|---|
| 1. | Patients who have been diagnosed as having diabetes have been recorded in the practice diabetes register. |
| 2. | The diagnosis of diabetes is correct (i.e. a patient labelled as being diabetic must have been shown to have diabetes). |
| 3. | The glycated haemoglobin has been checked at least annually and the result is within the normal range. |
| 4. | The records show that at least annually there has been an assessment of symptoms including hypoglycaemic attacks and general well-being. |
| 5. | The records show that at least annually the feet have been examined. |
| 6. | The records show that at least annually the patient's urine has been checked for albumin to detect early evidence of nephropathy. |
| 7. | The records show that at least annually the fundi have been examined for retinopathy through dilated pupils. |
| 8. | The records show that at least annually there has been an assessment of smoking habit. |
| 9. | The records show that at least annually the blood pressure has been checked and is within normal limits. |

| | 'Should do' |
|---|---|
| 10. | Each patient will be reviewed at regular intervals agreed with the patient (but not exceeding 12 months). |
| 11. | Each newly diagnosed patient (or their carer) will receive education about diabetes management. |
| 12. | The records show that at least annually the patient's diet has been reviewed. |
| 13. | The records show that at least annually the visual acuity has been checked. |
| 14. | The records show that at least annually the weight has been checked. |
| 15. | If the patient normally monitors the condition by urine or blood tests, the technique in performing the tests has been checked. |
| 16. | The records show that at least annually the patient's blood or urine monitoring records have been checked. |

| | 'Could do' |
|---|---|
| 17. | The records show that at least annually the blood lipids have been checked. |
| 18. | Information about complications of diabetes (retinopathy, nephropathy, neuropathy, amputations etc) is recorded on the diabetic register. |

## Findings

The findings are summarised in Tables A.15–19. Comparative information was available for most of the 'must do' criteria from an audit undertaken in Leicestershire involving 77 practices (Farooqi et al, 2000). The same audit protocol was used in this audit and the first data collection took place between 1994 and 1996. Therefore, the results provide a reasonable yardstick against which to compare the performance in Shipman's practice. In consequence, relevant information from the Leicestershire audit has been included in each Table, although it should be noted that only percentages were available for data about compliance with the criteria.

Shipman's practice provided care to a relatively high proportion of people with diabetes (Table A. 15) and had checked the glycated haemoglobin in a higher proportion, although the proportion whose diabetes was well controlled was slightly lower (Table A.16). Higher proportions of Shipman's patient had had their feet and blood pressure checked, although lower proportions had a record of checks of urine, fundi or smoking habits.

Comparative information was not available from the Leicestershire audit for the 'should do' or 'could do' criteria. However, many audits of care of people with diabetes have been undertaken in primary care and relevant data collated from such audits (Khunti et al, 1999) have been included in Tables A18 and 19 to provide a basis against which to compare the performance of Shipman's practice. In each of these audits, a group of general practices collected information about the care they had given to people with diabetes.

The percentages included in the Tables indicate the mean level of performance of the practices taking part in any particular audit. In order to illustrate the range of performance between audits, the lowest and highest percentages achieved in the audits are shown. The findings indicate that Shipman's practice compares well in reviewing patients, and checking weight and lipids, but less well in checking diet and visual acuity.

**Table A.15. Background information about people with diabetes included in the audit, including type of treatment and source of care. Data relate to Shipman's practice and a group of 77 practices in Leicestershire.**

| | Shipman's practice | | Leicestershire audit | |
|---|---|---|---|---|
| | number | % | number | % |
| **gender** | | | | |
| male | 17 | 56.7 | | |
| **treatment** | | | | |
| diet only | 5 | 16.7 | 1624 | 21.8 |
| oral hypoglycaemics | 12 | 40.0 | 3439 | 46.2 |
| insulin | 12 | 40.0 | 2264 | 30.4 |
| not known | 1 | 3.3 | 118 | 1.6 |
| **source of care** | | | | |
| general practice only | 21 | 70.0 | 4511 | 60.6 |
| hospital only | 2 | 6.7 | 783 | 10.5 |
| shared care | 4 | 13.3 | 1581 | 21.7 |
| not known | 3 | 10.0 | 480 | 6.4 |

**Table A.16. The numbers and percentages of patients whose care was in accordance with 'Must do' criteria 1-3, in Shipman's practice and a group of 77 practices in Leicestershire.**

| | Shipman's practice | | Leicestershire |
|---|---|---|---|
| | number | % | % |
| **Criterion 1** | | | |
| *recorded on register* | | | |
| yes | 29 | 96.7 | |
| **Criterion 2** | | | |
| *diagnosis correct* | | | |
| yes | 29 | 96.7 | |
| not clear | 1 | 3.3 | |
| **Criterion 3** | | | |
| *glycated Hb checked* | | | |
| yes | 27 | 90.0 | 82.0 |
| no | 1 | 3.3 | |
| not known | 2 | 6.6 | |
| *result of glycated Hb* | | | |
| normal | 10 | 37.0 | 45.1 |
| moderately raised | 15 | 55.6 | |
| poor | 2 | 7.4 | |

| | Shipman's practice | | Leicestershire |
|---|---|---|---|
| Table A.17. The numbers and percentages of patients whose care was in accordance with 'Must do' criteria 4–9, in Shipman's practice and a group of practices in Leicestershire. | | | |
| | number | % | % |
| **Criterion 4** | | | |
| *assessment of symptoms* | | | |
| yes | 9 | 30.0 | |
| not known | 21 | 70.0 | |
| | | | |
| **Criterion 5** | | | |
| *feet checked* | | | |
| yes | 22 | 73.3 | 65.6 |
| | | | |
| *if feet abnormal* | | | |
| normal | 18 | 60.0 | |
| advice | 2 | 6.7 | |
| refer chiropodist | 1 | 3.3 | |
| refer chiropodist and hospital | 1 | 3.3 | |
| | | | |
| **Criterion 6** | | | |
| *urine checked* | | | |
| yes | 5 | 16.7 | 65.3 |
| not known | 25 | 83.3 | |
| | | | |
| *urine abnormal* | 1 | | |
| | | | |
| **Criterion 7** | | | |
| *fundi checked* | | | |
| yes | 14 all by optometrist | 46.7 | 63.7 |
| no | 1 | 3.3 | |
| not known | 15 | 50.0 | |
| | | | |
| **Criterion 8** | | | |
| *smoking habits checked* | | | |
| yes | 1 | 3.3 | 68.2 |
| not known | 29 | 96.7 | |
| | | | |
| **Criterion 9** | | | |
| *BP checked* | | | |
| yes | 28 | 93.3 | 85.8 |
| no | 1 | 3.3 | |
| not known | 1 | 3.3 | |

**Table A.18. The numbers and percentages of patients whose care was in accordance with the 'Should do' criteria. Data from Shipman's practice and collated from audits undertaken by primary care audit groups.**

| | Shipman's practice | | Collated audits |
|---|---|---|---|
| | number | % | % |
| **Criterion 10** | | | |
| *review in past year* | 28 | 93.3 | 51.9–94.3 |
| yes | 2 | 6.7 | |
| no | | | |
| | | | |
| **Criterion 11** | | | |
| *education for new patients* | 9 | | |
| diagnosed in past 2 years & | 4 | 44.4 | |
| education recorded as given | | | |
| | | | |
| **Criterion 12** | | | |
| *diet reviewed* | 8 | 26.7 | 48.0–92.2 |
| yes | 22 | 73.3 | |
| not known | | | |
| | | | |
| **Criterion 13** | | | |
| *visual acuity checked* | 15 | 50.0 | 51.9–74.0 |
| yes | 1 | 3.3 | |
| no | 14 | 46.7 | |
| not known | | | |
| | | | |
| **Criterion 14** | | | |
| *weight checked* | 26 | 86.7 | 66.1–77.4 |
| yes | 2 | 6.7 | |
| no | 2 | 6.7 | |
| not known | | | |
| | | | |
| *weight raised* | 14 | 50.0 | |
| advice given | 10 | 71.4 | |
| refer dietician | 2 | 20.0 | |
| no action | 2 | 20.0 | |
| | | | |
| **Criterion 15** | | | |
| *Monitoring technique* | | | |
| monitors blood or urine, not | | | |
| known if technique checked | 7 | | |
| | | | |
| **Criterion 16** | | | |
| *monitoring records checked* | | | |
| yes | 27 | 90.0 | |
| no | 1 | 3.3 | |
| not known | 2 | 6.7 | |

**Table A.19. The numbers and percentages of patients whose care was in accordance with the 'Could do' criteria. Information from Shipman's practice and collated audits undertaken by primary care audit groups.**

| | Shipman's practice | | Collated audits |
|---|---|---|---|
| | number | % | % |
| **Criterion 17** | | | |
| *lipids checked* | | | |
| yes | 17 | 56.7 | 15.7–46.6 |
| no | 11 | 36.7 | |
| not known | 2 | 6.7 | |
| | | | |
| **Criterion 18** | | | |
| *complications* | | | |
| none | 25 | 83.3 | |
| retinopathy | 3 | 10.0 | |
| amputation | 1 | 3.3 | |
| retinopathy and neuropathy | 1 | 3.3 | |

## Conclusion

The qualifications made in relation to the review of the care of people with angina also apply to the review of people with diabetes. Some patients who had been cared for by Shipman will have left the practice since his arrest, and no conclusion can be made about the quality of care they had received. Furthermore, differences in recording habits may explain some of the differences in levels of compliance with particular criteria of care. However, the information available about the patients still registered with the practice is reassuring. The level of performance was comparable to the performance of other practices elsewhere in the UK. In relation to some criteria, performance was better than the comparison practices, and in relation to other criteria performance was not as good. One explanation for the satisfactory levels of performance is that much routine diabetes care in the practice was provided by members of the team following structured policies.

## References

Clinical Governance Research and Development Unit (1999). The collation of audit data for the Northern Effectiveness and Outcomes Network (NEON). Report on audits of antiplatelet use of aspirin. Leicester: Clinical Governance Research and Development Unit, Department of General Practice and Primary Health Care, University of Leicester.

Farooqi A, Khunti K, Sorrie R (2000). Does clinical audit improve care? Lessons for clinical governance from a district-wide primary care audit of diabetes. Journal of Clinical Governance 8:152–6.

GMC (2000). Confidentiality: Protecting and Providing Information. London: General Medical Council.

Khunti K, Baker R, Lakhani M (1995). Management of Angina in General Practice. Audit protocol CT7. Leicester: Eli Lilly National Clinical Audit Centre, Department of General Practice and Primary Health Care, University of Leicester.

Khunti K, Baker R, Rumsey M, Lakhani M (1999). Quality of care of patients with diabetes: collation of data from multi-practice audits of diabetes in primary care. Family Practice 16:54–59

Wilcox D, Webster J, Forrest D (1996). Secondary prevention of occlusive vascular disease using low dose (75–325mg) daily aspirin. *Audit Trends* 4:102–106.